DATE DUE

Nov 17, 2003	
DISCARDED	

PRINTED IN U.S.A.

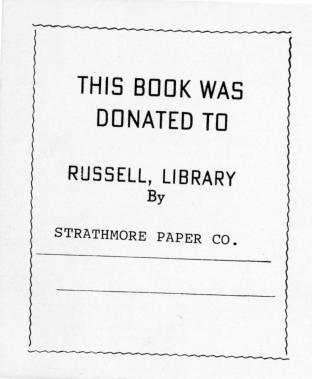

The DIABETES CURE

A Medical Approach That Can Slow, Stop, Even Cure Type 2 Diabetes

Vern S. Cherewatenko, M.D., and Paul Perry

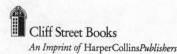

Cliff Street Books
An Imprint of HarperCollins*Publishers*

HarperCollins books may be purchased for educational, business, or sales promotional use. For information please write: Special Markets Department, HarperCollins Publishers, Inc., 10 East 53rd Street, New York, NY 10022.

FIRST EDITION

Designed by Nancy B. Field

Library of Congress Cataloging-in-Publication Data

Cherewatenko, Vern.
    The diabetes cure : a medical approach that can slow, stop, even cure type 2 diabetes / Vern Cherewatenko and Paul Perry.
       p.   cm.
    Includes index.
    ISBN 0-06-019210-0
    1. Non-insulin-dependent diabetes—Treatment.   2. Hydroxycitric acid—Therapeutic use.   3. Chromuim—Therapeutic use.   I. Perry, Paul. 1950–
II. Title.
RC662.18.C48   1999
616.4'6206—DC21   98-43193

---

99 00 01 02 03 ❖/RRD 10 9 8 7 6 5 4 3

I dedicate this book to Jeanine,
my wife and true soulmate,
and to our three beautiful and healthy girls,
Rachel, Kelsey, and Megan.

I love you, forever and always,

Dad

Contents

●●●●●●●●●●●

Disclaimer

Diabetes is a complicated and devastating disease. The material presented in this book is for patient education and informational purposes only. It is not meant to be a substitute for professional medical advice.

Diabetes is a disease that should be treated by a health care professional or a team of health care professionals with advanced training in diabetes.

Please discuss all aspects of *The Diabetes Cure* with your health care provider before using any of the information given here. It is important that you seek consultation with your health care provider before you change or alter any of the medications you may be taking.

The Diabetes Cure is a response to the request for a nonprescription, or natural, approach to diabetes mellitus, a disease that affects nearly 16 million people in the United States.

The evidence supports the conviction that increased understanding of diabetes, combined with an aggressive nutrition and exercise program enhanced by nutritional supplements, can have a pronounced and positive effect on those with type 2 diabetes mellitus.

The authors trust that the information in *The Diabetes Cure* will give patients a greater understanding of diabetes and the ability to increase compliance with a supervised medical program to control and cure type 2 diabetes. To "cure" is to apply a treatment, a drug, or another method to treat a medical problem. It means to restore the health of a patient with a disease or disorder or to obtain a favorable result by treating a disease or disorder. There is no overt or implied guarantee that the information presented here will benefit those with diabetes or those who may potentially become diabetic.

Acknowledgments

I would like to acknowledge the following people for assisting me to make this book more than just a vision:

My supportive wife, Jeanine, who bears the added responsibility of having a physician for a spouse, you are the wind beneath my wings. My children, Rachel, Kelsey, and Megan for all your hugs and finding the time to help me in so many ways. My coauthor, Paul Perry, a pillar of literary excellence. To Mel Morse, M.D., for introducing me to Paul and the staff of HarperCollins Publishers. To Diane Reverand, Editor and Publisher of Cliff Street Books, who endorsed the vision of helping educate people about such a severe disease. To Krista Stroever, who keeps it all happening, on time and on schedule, and Andrea Molitor, production editor, for her endless patience. To our agent, Nat Sobel, and his staff for handling the details. We also want to thank Mardy Fones for her editorial guidance. Without her fine work, this book would have taken far longer to produce.

A special thanks to my partner and colleague, David MacDonald, D.O., who has provided unyielding inspiration and assistance. To Dr. Soheyla Radfar, who has given so much of herself to teach a better way of living to me and others. To my dear friend James Coffin, for illustrating my life and providing wisdom's pearls. My medical colleagues, Kevin Connolly, Ph.D., C. J. DelMarco, D.O., Pieter de Wet, M.D., Steve Kaye, M.D., Chris Renna, D.O., Fred

Miser, M.D., Joan Robnett, Steve Hughes, M.D., Bev Kent, R.D., C.D., Nass Ordoubadi, M.D., Andy Abolins, M.D., Anthony Conte, M.D., Bill Downs at Interhealth, Howard Lyman, Jeff Bland, Ph.D., at HealthComm, for providing your medical expertise.

The strength and patience behind the scenes: Michael Pennington—"Superman," and business associates Larry Ream, Gregg Jordshaugen, Elaine Wilcox, and Ron Bozi. A special thank you to Gene Johnson, who went above and beyond. To Gwen Hoeck, my first employee, who has remained with me since residency. To the dedicated office staff, who has remained at my side, through all the challenges that face health care practitioners today. To my patients, who have remained flexible with my ever-changing schedule, your patience is a virtue. To those true friends . . . who no matter how long between talks . . . make me feel like I'm "home" again when we get together.

Last, but not least, to the patients who have diabetes mellitus, and to the dedicated researchers, organizations, doctors, and educators who are working toward curing this destructive disease.

Thank you all and please enjoy . . . *The Diabetes Cure!*

Introduction

"I'm sorry, you have diabetes."

These words are heard by 600,000 patients annually in the United States alone, and carry a dark cloud of despair. Not only will the patient suffer from this seemingly relentless disease, but so will family members. Diabetes is an expensive, troubling, and dangerous disease. Every year nearly 200,000 people die from diabetes, making it the seventh leading cause of death in the United States.

Diabetes is a disease characterized by high levels of glucose or sugar in the bloodstream. In type 2 or "age onset" diabetes, this high level of blood sugar is caused by the body's inability to use its own insulin to digest sugar. Medical researchers don't know why this happens and call it "Syndrome X." Poor nutrition, weight gain, and lack of exercise have contributed to type 2 diabetes's becoming one of the most prevalent health problems in the world. By early in the next century it is expected to reach worldwide epidemic proportions.

A person with diabetes runs the risk of a host of other problems, including blindness, heart disease, and strokes.

Some 15.7 million people, approximately 6 percent of the U.S. population, have diabetes, at a cost to treat of $105 billion per year. It is believed that 5.4 million adults in the United States have the disease and don't even know it.

How Chronic Illness Is Like Grief

Living day to day with a chronic illness like diabetes presents special challenges similar to the grieving process. You and the people around you may move through specific phases as you adjust to your illness and the demands it places on your body and life. Trying to avoid or ignore these feelings adds more stress, because it is only by moving through these phases that you can come to live a full, active life, despite diabetes.

The phases and the common response they elicit are:

- Shock and/or denial. "I don't really have diabetes. My diabetes isn't that bad. This isn't happening to me. None of those complications will happen to me. I don't feel sick, I feel fine."

- Anger. "It's the doctor's fault. I'm not going to follow this treatment plan and you can't make me. I have to die of something."

- Bargaining and/or negotiation. "I'll just have this extra helping now and make up for it tomorrow. If I exercise more, this will all go away."

- Depression and/or withdrawal. "I give up. It's hopeless. This disease is controlling my life."

- Acceptance. "It's hard work to stick with the program, but it's worth it."

After the initial denial and anger in reaction to this diagnosis, most patients will begin some type of behavior intervention, trying to undo years of nutritional, physiological, and even psychological abuse.

Though this is not the most exciting and upbeat start

to a book entitled *The Diabetes Cure*, the alarming statistics illustrate what those diagnosed with type 2 diabetes mellitus have to face. Diabetes mellitus is a disease of glucose imbalance. The disease is well described in the medical literature, and most physicians treat it daily in their practices. Much of this standard treatment is ineffective and passive. During the typical diabetic visit the doctor reviews the symptoms and runs a few tests. In laissez-faire fashion, the patient is told he or she is doing well, or needs to continue to improve in one area or another. Seldom does the physician give the patient the education and information necessary to *cure* or reverse diabetes.

Type 2 diabetes is an eminently curable disease. I know, because I have cured it in myself.

My brush with diabetes began when I was an eighteen-year-old premedical student. Leaving high school at six feet tall and 167 pounds, I entered the premedical program at Montana State University in Bozeman. My goal was to become a well-rounded family physician. I became "well-rounded," but not in the way I had originally intended.

The strenuous exercise of high school gave way to an exercise routine that amounted to carrying twenty pounds of books to and from classes. Many days I sat in my dorm room studying, while my friends engaged in serious exercise on the playing fields. It seemed as though everyone but me was outside playing softball or Frisbee, or chasing the opposite sex across the commons.

Along with strenuous study came strenuous eating. My interest in food stayed higher than my interest in exercise and fitness. I gained weight and ignored it or denied it. The person I saw in the mirror didn't look *that* heavy, I told myself. When my pants stopped fitting, I blamed it on the hot dryer instead of those hot beef sandwiches I was eating every day.

Throughout my premed studies, I worked at the local ambulance service as an emergency medical technician, which provided a broad exposure to a full spectrum of disease and injury. Many patients who had congestive heart failure, renal failure, blindness, and removed appendages were actually patients in the final stages of uncontrolled diabetes mellitus. Little did I know, as a budding doctor, that these patients were representative of my own future.

When I went off to medical school, I didn't leave my habits behind. I was still eating like a linebacker and exercising like a snail when I walked in the doors of the University of Washington medical school.

During Christmas break I decided to return to the emergency room to see the nurses I had befriended. I hadn't seen them in four months and wanted to let them know that I was firmly ensconced in medical school. I was anxious for them to meet the new man I was becoming.

I ran across the parking lot to the ER entrance on a bitter cold night. A small ache in my knee was barely noticeable as the large electric doors opened. The smell of alcohol and Betadine reminded me I was home.

After a quick hello to the ER doctor on call and a high five to the janitor, I saw one of my favorite nurses turn around. It had been four months since I had seen Jill, and I stood there with my arms up, waiting for her to hug me. As she turned around, her bright smile quickly turned into a puzzled frown.

"What happened to you?" she demanded.

My delight disappeared. There was nowhere to hide. I caught sight of myself in one of the hallway windows and couldn't deny that I had changed. I was forty pounds heavier than I had been when I left for med school. I had gained ten pounds per month.

Jill continued to talk to me, but all I could hear in my mind was the classic quote from Luke: "Physician, heal thyself."

The sad thing was that I didn't heal myself, not right away. at any rate. I continued to gain weight until I weighed 318 pounds, and then I did something about it. I had been diagnosed with borderline diabetes and given a glucose control drug to lessen the effects of glucose imbalance. On my own, I began to diet, exercise, take vitamins and minerals, and even experiment with the herb hydroxycitric acid, which I would eventually prescribe to patients in my own practice. After several months of hard work and behavioral change, I cured my own diabetes. I have never taken a glucose control medication again.

One of the ironies in my situation was that none of my professors at medical school ever told me I could cure diabetes. And, of course, no one researched the benefits of herbal remedies on type 2 diabetes. Instead they were tightly focused on the art of giving medicine.

During the last eight years I have been a practicing family physician in Renton, Washington. I have had the privilege of caring for many patients afflicted with diabetes—borderline diabetes, advanced diabetes, and complicated diabetes—and for patients who didn't know they had or would get diabetes. There are many people in this latter category.

The national diabetic prevention trial, one of the largest diabetes screening and research projects ever, has uncovered the shocking fact that there are three times more diabetics or "glucose intolerant" people than have been detected. This is an alarming statistic with potentially dangerous implications if the condition is not aggressively combated. The complications of diabetes are devastating and affect nearly every organ of the body.

Diabetes not only can destroy a human life but affects the people around the diabetic patient, who know that diabetes is a disease of lifestyle but maybe don't know to change lifestyle habits to make their loved one healthier. Although some people are living with diabetes very effectively and managing their diabetes well, many are not. They are frustrated and searching for information that will allow them to launch a successful and sustained attack against their diabetes.

The goal of this book is to give people with diabetes the information they need. By following a nine-point program that combines the standard tools of diabetes control and prevention—exercise, diet, stress reduction, and vitamin supplementation—with a mineral called chromium and an herb called HCA, you can prevent, control, and even cure type 2 diabetes. I emphasize the prevention aspects of the nine-point program because type 2 diabetes is one of the most preventable of all diseases. By following the nine-point program *before* you have diabetes, you can reduce your chances of getting type 2 diabetes and a host of other diseases of lifestyle, including heart disease and strokes. The cliché "Prevention is the best medicine" is repeated often because it is true.

The herbal portion of this nine-point program, HCA, is technically known as hydroxycitric acid, a readily available substance found in the brindle berry (*Garcinia cambogia*) and other Asian fruits. HCA reduces cravings for sweets and enhances the effectiveness of the body's own insulin. Used for years as an herbal alternative to diet drugs, HCA allows the muscles of the body to absorb more glucose, the sugar in the bloodstream that is the body's main form of fuel. The chromium taken with the HCA also helps with the absorption of glucose by the muscles.

The use of glucose is important. Glucose that is not used by the muscles and other body tissues stays in the bloodstream and causes the dangerous rise in blood sugar that is known as diabetes. Elevated blood sugar causes damage to the organs and other body parts.

In addition to increasing the rate of glucose absorption, hydroxycitric acid also binds up leftover glucose in the bloodstream, slowing down the rate at which carbohydrate is converted to fat. The result is a natural approach to glucose control, without side effects.

I discovered HCA while researching the scope of diet medications I could offer my weight-loss patients, many of whom are also diabetics. I found that combining lifestyle change with HCA allowed type 2 diabetics to go off medication almost immediately. For a natural approach to curing most cases of type 2 diabetes, HCA cannot be beat. Here are the reasons:

- **There are no side effects.** Unlike other diet drugs and the commonly used diabetes medications, there are no side effects to using hydroxycitrate. Indeed, one of its main source, the brindle berry, is commonly used as a flavoring in curry in many Asian countries. It is also used as a preservative and digestive aid. Researchers at Hoffmann–La Roche, the pharmaceutical company that has conducted a large amount of HCA research, consider hydroxycitrate to be safer than the citric acid in oranges and other citrus fruits.

- **HCA makes the body more receptive to insulin.** People with type 2 diabetes usually have sufficient insulin in their bloodstream to allow glucose into the muscles. It is the insulin resistance that prevents it from doing its job and letting the glucose enter and become energy. When that happens, people with insulin resistance overeat until there is so much glucose and insulin in their bloodstream that the glucose is pushed into the muscles. It is the body's inability to use insulin that makes so many type 2 diabetics overweight.

- **HCA keeps glucose stores high.** A study in the *American Journal of Clinical Nutrition* shows that HCA keeps the body from converting carbohydrates into fat. It also slows the formation of cholesterol and triglycerides, two known causes of heart disease and strokes.

- **HCA keeps the diabetic from getting hungry.** Research has shown that by keeping glucose stores high, this herb sends a message to the brain that the body is full and not hungry. This keeps the person with type 2 diabetes from gaining weight, which would make the diabetes even worse.

I have seen changes in my own patients as they have participated in our comprehensive, multidisciplinary diabetes and weight-management programs. They have learned through our Transitions Course the tools needed to make major lifestyle changes and keep these changes in effect.

The elements of the Transitions Course will be discussed throughout this book. We will help you understand the complicated inner working of your body and how various things you do affect its processes. With knowledge and understanding come compliance and control. The more you understand the information and knowledge we have about diabetes and how to prevent or cure it, the more compliant you will be with behavioral lifestyle changes, and the more control you will exert over your life. Our intent is to help you understand diabetes and develop new skills to control or prevent diabetes.

My patients have proven to me that diabetes can be controlled and cured. They have proven to me that the devastating effects of diabetes can be prevented, diverted, or reversed with much less effort than previously expected.

"Cure" is defined by the Webster's II Dictionary as "Recovery from illness. A course of medical treatment for restoring health. A remedy. To rid of." *The Diabetes Cure* is intended to do just that: to help you help yourself and others prevent or turn back this devastating disease.

VERN S. CHEREWATENKO, M.D., M.ED.
Seattle, WA

You may e-mail the author at:

drvern@healthmax.net

Or visit the Health*Max* Web site for more detailed information on associated programs and services at

http://www.healthmax.net

1

Can Diabetes Be Cured?

Diabetes is called the silent disease because it usually sneaks up on you without warning. It can start with feelings of overwhelming tiredness, or a need to eat even though you feel full to capacity. It sometimes shows up as blurry vision or as flashes of light. You might have a headache that lingers long past the aspirin you have taken to get rid of it, or a cut or sore that just doesn't heal.

Like most people, you will ignore these early signs by blaming them on stress or too little rest. After a while, the silent disease becomes too noisy to ignore. Perhaps you lose several pounds without being on a diet, or you have a numbness or tingling in your hands that makes you fear a stroke or tumor. You know something is wrong that should be attended to by a doctor.

After hearing your symptoms, the doctor suspects that you may have diabetes. Still, a diagnosis can't be made until at least a random plasma glucose test is done. This test is the simplest way to detect diabetes because it measures the amount of blood glucose in your system. It can be done without fasting to see if diabetes is possibly the problem. The nurse draws a vial of blood, and you wait for an answer from the laboratory.

The results aren't good. Your doctor tells you that the normal glucose count for this test is under 200 milligrams per deciliter (mg/dl). Your numbers, he explains are over 300.

"Could there be a mistake?" you ask, feeling a wave of fear.

"Possibly," says the doctor. "The random plasma glucose test tells us only that you might have diabetes. The fasting plasma glucose test tells us for sure if you do."

For the next eight hours you eat nothing before going back to the doctor for another blood test. "I hope it's different this time," says the nurse as she sticks the needle in your arm and draws a blood sample.

The next day you are back in an examining room with your doctor. She looks at the results of the blood test and begins to interpret them for you.

"In a patient without diabetes, the fasting glucose level will be less than 110 mg/dl," she says, looking down at your results. "You are substantially higher than that. I am afraid you have diabetes."

A weight seems to land on your shoulders as the news settles in. Diabetes. You don't know how it happened, you don't know when it started, and chances are you don't really know exactly what it is. But you do know that you have it and that it can be bad if you don't take care of it. You think about other people in your family who have developed diabetes at your age, and you remember how they have wrestled with the problem. You might even know someone who has become seriously impaired from this silent but deadly disease.

"I know this isn't good news, but millions of people have diabetes," says the doctor, trying to be reassuring.

"But I don't want diabetes," you say. "Can't you cure it?"

"Curing diabetes would take work on your part. Most patients aren't willing to do what it takes to cure diabetes.

On the other hand, I can treat it with drugs. The drugs I can give you will level out your blood sugar, but they won't cure diabetes, only treat it. You will have to take these drugs the rest of your life."

"But I don't want to be dependent on drugs the rest of my life," you say. "I am afraid of their side effects."

"All drugs have side effects," says your doctor. "But if you don't take them, you will suffer from the complications of diabetes, and those are much worse than the drugs to treat it."

The prospect of having to take drugs to survive is frightening. You trust your doctor, and you know that the treatment she is offering is the same one being used for other people with diabetes. You don't want to go down that slow road of degeneration that so many other people with diabetes have followed. You want to fight against your disease, but you just don't know how.

"Doctor, I am willing to do what it takes to cure my diabetes," you insist. "But tell me, can diabetes be cured?"

Battling "Syndrome X"

Can Diabetes Be Cured?

I have been asked this question many times by people who are facing a lifetime of diabetes drugs. The simple answer I give is a qualified yes. Type 2, or "age onset" diabetes, is usually considered a disease of lifestyle. Unlike type 1 diabetes, which usually begins before the age of twenty when the pancreas fails to produce insulin that the body needs to process energy, type 2 diabetes generally begins after the age of thirty and is caused by weight gain and physical inactivity. The combination of these two factors makes your muscles resistant to insulin, the hormone secreted by the pancreas that converts blood sugar, or glucose, into energy. Just as gasoline must be transported into the engine of a car for combustion to take place, glucose must be transported into your muscles for energy to be created. Insulin does that transporting.

FIGURE 1.1

The Pancreas

The pancreas is a large gland lying across the back of the abdominal wall. It has two secretions:

1. A digestive secretion poured into the duodenum.

2. A hormonal secretion passed into the bloodstream.

Capillaries drain the internal secretions of insulin and glucagon to the bloodstream to carry out their respective functions. It is the islets of Langerhans that produce the insulin in the body.

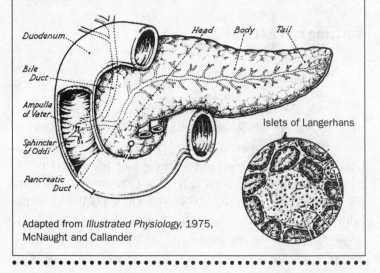

Adapted from *Illustrated Physiology*, 1975, McNaught and Callander

If your muscles are resistant to insulin, or your pancreas isn't creating enough insulin, glucose builds up in your blood, making it a thick sludge that is hard for the heart to circulate. Blood with too much glucose clogs arteries, causing heart attacks, strokes, and a number of other very serious problems. Muscles that can't use large enough quantities of glucose waste away as nerves that don't get glucose die.

The cause of insulin resistance isn't known and is called "Syndrome X," a name coined by Dr. Gerald Reaven of Stanford University.

In general terms, with Syndrome X the cells don't let insulin do its job, which is to "open up" the cells and let glucose enter and be used as energy. When this happens, the levels of glucose in the blood becomes higher and higher. Excess body fat and too little exercise combine to create Syndrome X. Sometimes the pancreas must work overtime to produce insulin. An overworked pancreas can become damaged, leading to an organ that fails to produce very much insulin at all. If that occurs, you might have to take artificial insulin.

Syndrome X is a double-edged sword. Not only is it the main cause of type 2 diabetes, it also causes you to gain weight, which makes the disease worse. Weight gain takes place when the lack of glucose in your cells blocks your satiety response to food, that feeling in your brain of being full and no longer wanting to eat. The feeling of satiety is related to the amount of glucose contained in your muscles and brain. If you are insulin-resistant, glucose takes longer to get into your brain's hunger centers, so you keep eating until it finally does. In the meantime, glucose reaches higher and higher levels in the bloodstream, which leads to the many symptoms and complications of diabetes.

Although some prescription medications have been very effective in normalizing glucose levels, they can also lead to sharp drops in glucose levels that force you to eat larger quantities of food. When that happens, you gain more weight and your condition becomes worse.

After you rely for years on prescription drugs for the treatment of type 2 diabetes, your disease generally becomes progressively more severe.

Waging War on Diabetes

Although allopathic medicine has done a good job of extending the life of diabetic patients, it has not done a good job of curing or preventing this disease. Many references in medical books declare that there is no cure for diabetes at this time. I attended one of the most prestigious medical schools in the country, and I never heard one of my professors say that diabetes could be cured.

The fact is that it can be cured. By taking the multidisciplinary approach outlined in this book, I and other doctors have been able to reduce diabetes patients' dependency on prescription drugs or eliminate the drugs altogether. In my program, I use a common weight-loss herb known as hydroxycitric acid, or HCA, which has been used for years as an herbal alternative to diet drugs like fen-phen and Redux.

HCA, unlike these controversial diet drugs that work by altering brain chemistry, allows the muscles of the body to absorb more glucose. When this happens, a "full" signal is sent to the brain, resulting in a reduced food intake.

In addition to increasing the rate of glucose absorption, hydroxycitric acid also binds up leftover glucose in the bloodstream, slowing down the rate at which glucose is converted to fat. The result is a natural approach to glucose control, without dangerous side effects.

A Natural Approach

I discovered HCA while researching the scope of diet medications I could offer my patients. As a bariatric physician, one who specializes in weight loss, I have treated more than 5,000 people for obesity. Many of these patients have type 2 diabetes and have taken diabetes medication for years.

When they come to my clinic, I start them on a comprehensive program that involves regular exercise, sensible eating, vitamin and mineral supplements, and medication to curb their appetite. I have had the opportunity to see the effects of virtually every diet drug ever marketed on type 2 diabetes. I have found that a combination of lifestyle change with any diet drug will allow a person with type 2 diabetes to eliminate medication or greatly reduce the amount needed almost immediately.

Why Not Diet Drugs?

The notion that diet drugs—like HCA or any other type— have an effect on type 2 diabetes might be hard to believe. Aren't these drugs aimed at making you lose weight by eating less?

The answer is yes. Since the drugs make you lose weight, they have other effects on the human body as well. Several studies have shown the positive effects of diet drugs on type 2 diabetes. For example, a 1995 double-blind study in New Zealand found that insulin sensitivity was dramatically increased in patients taking dexfenfluramine, a popular diet drug. This insulin sensitivity increased after only one week of therapy and before any weight loss.

Other studies have had the same results. Repeated controlled studies have shown "improved glycemic control" among people with type 2 diabetes through the use of diet drugs. Diet doctors have noted anecdotally that many of their patients with diabetes are able to stop or greatly reduce their use of type 2 medication within a week or two of starting diet drugs like Redux or fen-phen.

Of the thousands of patients treated in my clinics, many people with diabetes have gone medication-free as a result of taking diet drugs. In addition, insulin-dependent patients have been able to reduce the amount of insulin they take by as much as a third, just by taking diet drugs of all kinds, including HCA.

Medical science does not yet know the full effects of many diet drugs. Recent research has shown that these diet drugs may carry a substantial health risk. A Mayo Clinic study, for example, linked the diet drug fen-phen to heart disease in women, resulting in a warning against its use from the doctors who conducted the research. An article in a recent issue of *Hospital Practice* discussed the positive effects of diet drugs on type 2 diabetes, but then issued a warning to doctors who might consider prescribing them to patients. "Given the risks and caveats associated with anorectic drug therapy," the authors wrote, "one might wonder whether the potential benefits are worth the effort."

HCA, on the other hand, has no side effects. Ten years worth of research—both animal and human—shows that HCA reduces appetite by means of increased glycogen production. HCA also slows the process of converting carbohydrates into triglycerides, a form of blood fat that is linked to a higher incidence of heart disease and strokes. Here is more research showing the effect of HCA on the causes of type 2 diabetes:

- In an eight-week, double-blind study, fifty obese volunteers were placed on a low-fat diet. Twenty-nine of the patients were given HCA before each meal, while the rest were given a placebo. After eight weeks the HCA group lost an average of eleven pounds per person, while the placebo group lost an average of only four pounds per person. The reason given for the added weight loss was greater appetite suppression caused by increased insulin sensitivity.

- Rats fed a high-fat diet supplemented with HCA were compared with rats fed a high-fat diet not supplemented with HCA. After fifteen days the HCA group ate less, lost weight, and had lower levels of serum triglycerides than the other group. Much of the effect was attributed to the fact that increased insulin sensitivity reduces appetite.

- In two human trials published in *The Bariatrician*, patients were asked to assess their level of energy after one group was given HCA and another group was given a placebo. The group that were given HCA consistently reported more energy than the group given the placebo. All were then blood-tested. The HCA group had far lower levels of blood sugar than the placebo group, indicating that the blood sugar had been absorbed into their systems.

A Case Study

A number of studies show the effectiveness of HCA in weight loss, reduction of blood serum cholesterol and triglycerides, and—most important for the person with diabetes—ability to increase insulin sensitivity. But there is no greater test of a drug than seeing it in action in a patient.

Typical of the cases I have seen is a man I'll call Jim, an overweight forty-three year-old with a fasting glucose level of 176 mg/dl, which put him well into the blood sugar range for type 2 diabetes.

Jim's diabetes was not his only concern. Other tests found that he was also at risk for cardiovascular disease. His cholesterol level was 356—156 points higher than the ideal recommended by the American Heart Association. Triglycerides were a whopping 990, more than 700 points higher than the ideal. Numbers like these guaranteed that Jim's diabetes would worsen and cardiovascular disease would develop.

I put Jim on 1,000 milligrams of HCA, one capsule before each meal. He was also put on a low-fat diet and an exercise routine that had him walking between thirty minutes and an hour per day.

In less than two weeks he was tested again. His glucose level had dropped to 111, well within normal. Also, total cholesterol was reduced to 262. The most amazing reduction was his triglyceride level, down almost 600 points, to 396.

During the next two months Jim's numbers continued to drop. At his most recent checkup his glucose level was 85. His cholesterol level continued to drop to 185, and his triglyceride level to 117. With numbers like that, it was not only Jim's diabetes that was being reversed. Jim's blood composition was in a range that could actually *reverse* cardiovascular disease that might have occurred from years of high cholesterol and borderline diabetes.

A Rising Problem

The most startling aspect of this case study is not that Jim was able to cure his diabetes. For me, it was his age—forty-three. Since 1958 the number of Americans who have been diagnosed with diabetes has increased six-fold. According to the Centers for Disease Control and Prevention, another 6 million people are unaware that they have the disease. Other studies place that figure even higher, estimating that half of adult diabetics are undiagnosed.

More people worldwide have diabetes than ever before. A recent estimate puts the global number of people with type 2 diabetes at 120 million. In addition, more of those people with diabetes are younger than ever before. More than 10 million of the known 15 million type 2 diabetes in America are baby boomers, born between 1946 and 1964. A growing number are children, a frightening scenario since there are no studies to guide us on how to provide safe treatment. Since type 2 diabetes in children is such a recent phenomenon, we have not yet conducted any studies.

What is causing this sudden and catastrophic rise in type 2 diabetes? The answer is poor diet and lack of exercise. The high-fat diet of the West has been adopted worldwide, with fatty fast foods replacing the rice- and vegetable-based diets that used to dominate in many countries. Along with diets higher in fat has come a more sedentary lifestyle. Like Americans, most people in the world don't do as much

BOX 1.1

WARNING! WARNING!

The CDC has announced in 1998 the following statistics:

- More diabetes than ever is surfacing in the U.S.
- Nearly 16 million cases, of which one-third are undiagnosed.
- Since 1980, diabetes has increased in all age groups.
- Diabetes has increased especially in the black population.
- The CDC recommends an urgent need to prevent diabetes and the complications of diabetes.
- The International Diabetes Institute issued a statement cautioning that type 2 diabetes apprears to be an epidemic in many regions of the world.
- They felt that by the year 2010, the cases of type 2 diabetes will double.
- This will increase the worldwide total from 123 million people to 220 million people afflicted with type 2 diabetes.

More information regarding the statistical updates by the CDC is available on their Web site at: www.cdc.gov/diabetes

physical work or play as they used to. This lack of proper diet and exercise has led to obesity, which is present in 95 percent of people with type 2 diabetes.

The number of people with diabetes who don't know they have the disease has alarmed the medical community to such an extent that massive screenings have been suggested by some researchers to stave off "the beginning of an epidemic."

History of the Mystery

It has been only in this century that the causes and treatment of diabetes have been known. Before that, it was a mysterious disease, the cause of which was only a guess.

The earliest known record of diabetes discussed frequent urination or "polyuria" as a symptom, on papyrus written by Hesy-Ra, a Third Dynasty Egyptian physician. During the first century A.D., Arateus described diabetes as "the melting down of flesh and limbs into urine" and Galen of Pergamum, a Greek physician, felt diabetes was a form of kidney failure.

The diagnosis of diabetes was frequently confirmed by "water tasters," who sensed the sweet taste of the urine by drinking it. The term *mellitus* is derived from the Latin word for "honey." Diabetes mellitus was used to describe the disease of sweet urine.

Early in the nineteenth century urine testing became more scientific when the first chemical tests of the urine were developed to measure sugar levels. The French physician Priorry recommended high doses of sugar as a diabetes treatment during the late 1850s. Twenty years later Bouchardat, another French physician, reported that excess glucose in the urine disappeared in his diabetes patients during the Franco-Prussian War food rationing program.

Claude Bernard in the nineteenth century researched glucose metabolism in the liver and studied the physiology of the pancreas. His research began the increased scientific study of the relationship of the pancreas and glucose metabolism. Later in that century Italian diabetes physician Catoni locked up patients to modify their diets.

In 1869 a devoted German medical student revealed

his research on a two-cell system in the pancreas. One set of cells, he believed, secreted digestive juices, and the other set had an unknown function. The student's name was Paul Langerhans, and the two cell types produced insulin and became known as the "islets of Langerhans." Twenty years after Langerhans described the two cell types, Minkowski and von Mering, a pair of researchers in Austria, surgically removed the pancreas from a dog to examine the effects and related biological changes.

The first "fad diets" came on the scene in the early 1900s; these included eating an abundance of single items such as potatoes, rice, oatmeal, or milk and were largely unsuccessful. George Zuelzer of Germany gave the first injections of "pancreatic extract" in 1908, which resulted in many severe side effects.

During the later part of 1920 through 1922, Dr. George Banting researched, developed, and tested pancreatic extracts for their effectiveness on diabetes.

On May 21, 1922, James Havens became the first American to receive insulin successfully. Treatment of diabetes became more widespread when Eli Lilly and Company began to manufacture insulin. Banting and Macleod received the Nobel Prize for Medicine in 1923.

Further research in the 1940s provided insight into the relationship of diabetes to other diseases, namely kidney disease and eye degeneration. The insulin syringe was developed in 1944, and the first oral medications for diabetes were seen in 1955 to help patients lower blood sugar levels. Type 1 diabetes and type 2 diabetes were recognized as separate syndromes in 1959, with type 1 dependent on insulin and type 2 not dependent on insulin.

Patient education expanded in the 1960s with American Diabetes Association recommendations to test urine at home to increase glucose control. Public awareness is beginning to grow as results of the Diabetes Prevention Program, research which has determined that there are a great number of undiagnosed people with diabetes, and efforts are under way to identify them.

Why Alternative Therapy?

For years the notion of using alternative therapy to treat type 2 diabetes has been surpassed by the use of medications. It seems as though every year has at least one new treatment for diabetes. One of the most recent, Rezulin, was pulled from the European market when patients died and studies showed that it had side effects that were dangerous to the liver.

Many people have relied on drugs and little more to treat their disease. They have mistakenly thought that glucose-control drugs alone can bring them back to normal. Don't get me wrong, the glucose-control drugs discussed in the next chapter are great, but they have side effects that can include a worsening of the disease. Although they are prescribed for almost everyone with type 2 diabetes, they are not necessarily for everyone.

More and more people with diabetes are looking for an approach to their disease that has no side effects and gives them the possibility of curing diabetes with a natural method that actually makes them healthier.

In the last several years I have seen an increase in the demand for alternative treatments as patients realize that many drugs just conceal the disease process and don't really slow or stop it. These patients are the ones who are willing to do more than simply take a pill. Pills alone won't do it. Even the most powerful of the diabetes drugs can't stop diabetes if the patient will not implement the lifestyle changes necessary to control glucose levels.

That is why the Diabetes Cure requires more than just a few tablets of HCA per day. The prescription that I am writing with this book calls for a multidisciplinary approach to glucose control involving:

- Daily HCA.
- Thirty minutes to an hour a day of enjoyable exercise.
- Monitoring the type and amount of food you eat.
- Daily vitamin and mineral supplementation— especially chromium—to add punch to your body's metabolism and defenses.
- Daily stress reduction that gives you time for yourself and gives your body time to regroup.

Each of these aspects of the Diabetes Cure will be covered in detail in the pages ahead. Much of this is information that should have been given to you clearly and carefully when you found out about your disease. Chances are, it wasn't. Doctors today have less time for patients because managed care has forced them to spend more time on business. Studies have shown that the average doctor spends seven minutes completing paperwork for every one minute spent with a patient. This patient-to-paperwork ratio has had a direct effect on patient education, which is time-consuming. With little time to spare, doctors are prescribing diabetes medications and sending their patients out the door when they should be helping them make the necessary lifestyle changes.

Many in the medical community are concerned about this reliance on medication at the cost of patient education. In *Clinical Diabetes,* a medical journal published by the American Diabetic Association, editor Alan J. Garber, M.D., Ph.D., expressed the concern of those of us who believe in a more holistic approach to this disease.

> Managed care organizations until recently generally have not espoused the commitment to patient education required to make diet and exercise a meaningful prescription. Physicians have all too willingly participated in the prescription-writing frenzy that is often necessary to control Type 2 diabetes. . . .
>
> Thus, the recent proliferation of effective oral therapies is both a blessing and a curse. It is a blessing for patients who are actively attempting to care for their diabetes and for the physicians who participate in such efforts. But it may be a curse for patients who can delude themselves and their physicians that such agents are effective even in the absence of diet and exercise, points which have not been demonstrated in prospective, randomized, clinical trials.

It's Up to You!

At its very heart, *The Diabetes Cure* is about taking charge of your own disease. By educating yourself with the information in this book, you can slow, stop, or even cure your type 2 diabetes.

Most people respond to a diagnosis of diabetes by becoming depressed. Not only do they have a fear of the unknown, but they also fear "making a mistake" that will raise their glucose levels and cause damage. There is, of course, reason to fear diabetes. It can be a relentless disease that chips away at your weak spots and causes complications like heart disease, vision problems, and strokes. On the other hand, knowledge and understanding of this disease can put control back into your life.

Of course, taking the holistic road and trying to cure a disease is harder than just managing it. When patients express doubt about their ability to change their lifestyle rather than rely on the false security of medication, I ask them to answer three question for themselves.

- If not this, what?
- If not you, who?
- If not now, when?

Good luck as you begin the transformation that will give you control over your disease.

2

Fighting a Winning Battle

A patient came to me with the frustration felt by many people with diabetes. Phil had been diagnosed more than four years earlier with type 2 diabetes. His doctor had given him a drug that would increase the amount of insulin produced by his pancreas. Although he had plenty of insulin circulating in his blood already, his cells had become resistant to insulin. By increasing the amount of insulin, the drug forced the cells to open up to insulin and let the glucose in to be used as energy.

This medication worked fine for about a year. Then Phil began to notice that he had gained a considerable amount of weight. Concerned about the dangers of gaining weight, he asked his doctor for help and was given information about diet and exercise, the first time he remembered hearing about either one in relation to his disease.

He was fairly diligent in following the advice, although he admitted that he did not exercise every day and frequently "fell off the wagon" when it came to eating right. Still, he was gaining weight and not feeling so good, either. Some of his symptoms were returning. He would have periods of binge eating that he just could not avoid.

Over the course of three years he had gained more than thirty pounds. This shocked him. Although he had always been a little on the heavy side, he had never gained weight as rapidly as he did when he started his medication for diabetes. When his physician increased the amount of medication he was taking in hopes of getting rid of some of his symptoms, Phil began to feel even worse. At times he felt literally driven to the refrigerator by feelings of hypoglycemia, or low blood sugar. He was also experiencing extraordinary thirst.

The return of Phil's diabetes symptoms led his doctor to increase his dosage of medication. If his symptoms worsened, Phil's doctor said he might add another medication to boost the effectiveness of the one he was already getting. If Phil's problems continued to worsen, the doctor told him he might be forced to add an injection of insulin to his daily medication regimen.

Phil's concern that his condition was not improving led him to me. I had treated a friend of his for obesity, which also led to curing his borderline diabetes, the early stages before type 2 diabetes is diagnosed.

I had him follow the Diabetes Cure to the letter, with particular emphasis on exercise and stress reduction. After administering the 11–11 Scale contained in chapter 7 (page 183), on stress reduction, I could tell that he needed relief from several stressors in his life. I did not take him off his medication, since a person with diabetes should never stop medication "cold turkey." Rather, I started him on daily doses of HCA and chromium and had him watch his glucose carefully.

Within three months he had lost close to ten pounds and was feeling free of symptoms. I was gradually able to wean him from his medication until he was taking about half as much as he had when he first came to see me.

Phil has continued to improve, and the longer he follows the steps in the diabetes cure, the more he will improve. He now realizes two very important things about diabetes:

- It is a proactive disease, one you must fight constantly on every front.
- Diabetes drugs do not cure the disease and were never intended to. Taken alone, they can only slow the progression of this relentless disease.

Symptoms, Not Cause

Historically, diabetes treatment has been aimed at treating the symptoms of the disease and not its cause. That means the goal of most diabetes drugs is to prevent the problems diabetes causes, like excess thirst, hunger, urination, irritability, weakness, and fatigue. They do relieve these symptoms, but they do it without making the body more receptive to insulin, which is the cause of 95 percent of all cases of type 2 diabetes.

This is the best that most diabetes drugs can do. Most of these drugs work by increasing the amount of insulin in your blood, slowing the release of glucose by your liver, or slowing the absorption of food by your intestines. Since they do not increase insulin sensitivity, these drugs alone will not win the war. They will only help you fight a losing battle.

People with diabetes who rely heavily on drugs generally do not have good glucose control. Every time glucose moves into the danger zone (above 200 mg/dl), more damage is done to the body, and complications are more likely to arise.

This was proven in the Diabetes Control and Complications Trial (DCCT), a ten-year National Institutes of Health study of glucose control in people with diabetes, mentioned earlier. Their study showed that hyperglycemia, or high blood sugar, leads to nerve and vascular damage that can increase the risk of eye, nerve, and kidney disease. The good news is that careful blood glucose control through an intensive regimen of diet and exercise reduced the risk of complications by 50 to 75 percent.

The Diabetes Drugs

Physicians have five different "classes" of prescription drugs to treat type 2 diabetes. All have side effects, and none can be relied upon alone. They all require a multidisciplinary approach to fighting diabetes. Without incorporating at least diet and exercise as part of your treatment, you are fighting a losing battle against a disease that never rests, no matter how powerful the drug is that your doctor has prescribed.

Sulfonylureas. This long-standing class of drugs has been the mainstay of the oral medications for many years. **Micronase** and **Diabeta** are two of the more popular sulfonylureas.

These drugs stimulate the pancreas, increasing the amount of insulin that is secreted into the bloodstream. This added insulin forces the glucose into the muscles like a chemical battering ram.

The problem with sulfonylureas is that they don't improve your insulin sensitivity; rather they increase the amount of insulin in the blood. This solves the short-term problem by lowering your blood glucose levels, but it creates long-term problems by encouraging weight gain. This drug increases insulin, but some type 2 patients have insulin levels *five times* above normal levels already.

The process of increasing insulin levels leaves many people with diabetes hypoglycemic. As a result, the sudden drop in blood sugar that this class of drug causes compels them to eat. People with hypoglycemia get such symptoms of low blood sugar as mental confusion, dizziness, and even loss of consciousness.

The result of hypoglycemia is overeating, which leads to weight gain, which leads to increasingly poor insulin sensitivity. This is precisely opposite the effect we want to see. People with diabetes should lose those unnecessary pounds, not accumulate more!

Sulfonylureas are known to increase cholesterol and triglyceride levels, both of which are linked to heart disease.

There are currently seven sulfonylureas to choose from, three of which are improved or "second-generation" drugs. These latest offspring are **glyburide, glipizide,** and **glimepiride**.

Biguanides. Developed in 1994, biguanides approach glucose control from the opposite direction from sulfonylureas. Rather than increase the amount of insulin coming from the pancreas, they slow the amount of glucose entering the blood from the liver and the small intestines where food is digested.

The biguanides are an improvement over the sulfonylureas, because they do not cause weight gain or increase the risk of heart disease. They also have been shown to increase the levels of HDL or "good" cholesterol while lowering triglyceride levels.

The benefits of this medication have their cost. People taking biguanides report bloating, nausea, cramps, abdominal fullness, and diarrhea. People with heart, liver, or kidney problems are discouraged from taking this medication.

Typical of the biguanides is **metformin**.

Alpha-glucosidase inhibitors. The alpha-glucosidase inhibitors, like **acarbose** and **precose**, slow the breakdown of starch in the small intestines by interfering with the alpha-glucosidase enzyme. This enzyme is responsible for breaking down food into glucose. When the enzyme's action is blocked, a rise in blood glucose levels is prevented.

Although effective in blocking glucose, it can cause some unfriendly side effects. Excessive gas and flatulence, accompanied by diarrhea and abdominal pain, make it a potential source of social accidents. These symptoms make it a drug that should be avoided by people with irritable bowel disease, ulcers, and colitis.

Elevated liver function can also occur with acarbose, making it dangerous for people with liver problems.

Thiszolidinediones. The newest class of diabetes drug is perhaps the most controversial. Brand-named **Rezulin**, this drug is the first on the market to help the body make better use of its insulin by stimulating receptor sites in tissue, the "doorways" through which glucose passes from the blood.

Some studies have tested the use of Rezulin with sulfonylureas. Although it lowered the average glucose levels, patients in one study had still gained 5.8 to 13.1 pounds one year after starting the medication.

Although Rezulin improves insulin sensitivity, it is not a magic bullet, and it is not without side effects. Like other medications used to treat type 2 diabetes, it has serious risks. Cases of liver problems have been reported, including fatality, which led to the drug being banned in Europe. For this reason, patients are required to undergo regular liver function tests. Headaches have also been reported, along with infections and general pain.

Meglitinides. A blood-glucose-lowering agent that is derived from benzoic acid, these drugs cause an increased release of insulin by the pancreas. Brand-named **Prandin** or **Repaglinide**, the meglitinides stop acting much more quickly than the sulfonylureas, which minimizes any hypoglycemic effects.

Weight gain has been associated with meglitinides, along with the lowering of white blood cells and platelets and an increase in liver enzymes.

Insulins—new and old. Insulin is always used with type 1 diabetes, since people with that form of the disease do not produce insulin of their own. With type 2 diabetes, insulin is used as a last resort.

About 29 percent of people with type 2 diabetes are eventually treated with insulin. Treatment of type 2 diabetes with insulin could usually be avoided with adherence to good diet and exercise routines. Although diabetes educators do a very good job in educating patients who need insulin, it is often information that arrives too late. By the time many patients find out they need insulin, they are often less motivated to make the changes called for to reverse their condition. They have given up, and are willing to accept that their diabetes will be fought by medication only.

Insulin, available since 1922, is designed either to act quickly or to act several hours after administration. Whether short- or long-acting, insulin tells the liver to stop producing glucose and to start using it. In addition, insulin tells the muscles to suck in glucose and to start burning it for fuel. Insulin can also tell the fat cells to take in glucose, but this occurs to a lesser degree.

Insulin dosage and timing have profound effects on the blood glucose levels. Too much, and the blood glucose level falls, leading to hypoglycemia. Too little insulin, and there is not enough to drive the glucose into the cells that need it. Insulin can be used by people with type 2 diabetes with or without some of the oral medications. Usual doses of insulin are given two times a day, morning and evening, to try to keep the glucose levels at or near normal range.

The delicate balance between such factors as food intake, energy expenditure through exercise, medication dosages, illness, and stress all interact to raise or lower the levels of glucose in the blood. The closer the blood glucose levels stay to the normal range, the fewer systemic effects diabetes will have.

As wonderful as insulin is, it has side effects like all diabetes medications. Hypoglycemia, weight gain, and rapid occurrence of blood vessel disease are all potential side effects of insulin therapy. These side effects make it necessary to have close supervision by a health care provider trained in diabetes when undergoing insulin treatment.

So What Is HCA?

The plant kingdom has always been a medicine chest for humans. For millions of years nature was the only place we could go for medicine. Even today, more than 30 percent of our medications are derived from plants. Among the drugs that have come from the plant kingdom is aspirin, which was first found contained in willow bark as far back as ancient Greece. Another common drug, reserpin, was found in plants and is now used to treat high blood pressure and congestive heart failure. Digitalis, used to treat cardiac arrhythmias, was refined from the foxglove plant.

It is estimated that approximately 80 percent of the world's population uses herbal medicines, many because they prefer a more gentle and natural approach to treatment.

Among the thousands of plants used effectively is a reddish fruit the size of a small orange from the botanical tree *Garcinia cambogia*. When this rind is dried and ground into powder, it has uses for many different diseases. In India, for instance, garcinia is sometimes used as a topical application for infections. It also has use as a "chewing stick" to keep teeth and gums healthy. In some countries it is used as an aphrodisiac and even as a treatment for parasites and liver problems. In China, herbalists give garcinia to patients with type 2 diabetes and heart problems.

It was the use of *Garcinia cambogia* in traditional treatments that led to an interest in its essence by researchers. Chemical researchers knew that it worked as a treatment for a variety of conditions, but they didn't know why. In 1965 two researchers found that the active ingredient in this herbal remedy was hydroxycitric acid

(HCA), and research on its effects began. What they found with HCA was a chemical compound that did more than expected.

A chemist at Brandeis University, J. A. Watson, Ph.D., found by surprise that hydroxycitrate would trick cells into not synthesizing fat. If cells could not synthesize fat, they would not store fat, which meant there would be less buildup of fat in the liver and on the body.

Several rat studies were undertaken in the 1970s to confirm Watson's findings. Researchers at Brandeis University and at Hoffmann–La Roche Laboratories used rats to demonstrate that HCA reduced the synthesis of fat in living animals. They then began to speculate that HCA might have uses as a weight-control drug.

Researchers Ann Sullivan and Joseph Triscari fed HCA to test animals in their regular diet and found that they did not gain weight as fast as another group of test animals fed the same amount of food. Further examination of the test animals led them to the realization that HCA blocks fat accumulation.

In simple terms, HCA blocks fat synthesis by interfering with part of the Krebs cycle, the chemical process by which our cells convert energy into fuel. When food is eaten in greater quantities than our bodies need on any given day, the extra energy is converted into fat. HCA disrupts the cycle that converts this energy into fat, causing the excess energy to be stored as glycogen instead of absorbed on thighs and other places.

Further Discovery

Further animal research led to another discovery: Rats that were fed HCA became satiated or "full" on less food than the control group. They ate less food because the HCA made them less hungry. Further study of the animals told the researchers why satiety was reached so quickly. The rate of *gluconeogenesis*—food converted to glucose by the liver—was nearly doubled in the animals fed HCA. When the amount of glucose in the liver is high, it signals the brain through the vagus nerve that it needs no more food, and the person stops eating.

Additional research on animals found that HCA probably increases the metabolic rate and speeds the burning of fat by the liver.

All these factors—lower synthesis of fat, satiation or becoming "full" on less food, and speeding the burning of fat by the liver—can have an extremely positive effect on people with type 2 diabetes.

Further animal research led to another finding that might be the most important factor of all in the control of type 2 diabetes: HCA greatly reduced the amount of fatty acids in the bloodstream. In some studies animals that were fed a combination of HCA and a high-fat diet had one-third the levels of fatty acids as rats fed the high-fat diet only.

Lower blood fats are particularly important to people with type 2 diabetes, since some researchers speculate that elevated levels of free fatty acids like triglycerides and LDL cholesterol can lead to insulin insensitivity, that "Syndrome X" referred to earlier that causes the disease.

Research into HCA has been halted by Hoffmann–La Roche because, in my opinion, the drug company could not patent an extract of a natural product.

Other Research

Despite the lack of funding from drug companies, research into the effects of HCA have continued. Its effects on body weight, blood lipids, insulin sensitivity, and satiety—all of which are important factors in the control and cure of type 2 diabetes—have continued to be evaluated. When it comes to altering the factors that lead to type 2 diabetes, HCA passes the test.

An eight-week study examined fifty-four people who had the risk factors for diabetes (overweight, inactive, poor blood lipid profile). Twenty-two of these subjects took HCA before each meal, and the remainder were given a placebo. After eight weeks, the study group had lost an average of 11.1 pounds per person while the placebo group lost 4.2 pounds per person.

The HCA group had an easier time making recommended lifestyle changes, including eating a diet low in fat and following a daily regimen of sensible exercise, probably because the HCA left them feeling "full" after eating less food.

The HCA group also had a marked decrease in serum cholesterol and triglycerides. They also reported a higher level of energy, possibly caused by an increase in insulin sensitivity.

Three medications were tested on 128 patients over an eight-week period. Two of the groups were given two different diet drugs that did not contain HCA. The third group was given a medication containing HCA. The twenty-nine subjects in the HCA group lost an average of 11.48 pounds per person, while the other two groups lost 9.52 and 6.65 pounds per person respectively.

Hunger levels were significantly lower in the HCA group, as were lipid levels. Energy levels were higher, however.

Volunteers were given HCA for eight weeks to study its effects on obesity, a major risk factor of type 2 diabetes. The study group consisted of sixty women and fifteen men who weighed from 135 to 253 pounds and varied in age from twenty-one to sixty-five years of age. The 250 milligrams daily dosage of HCA, taken thirty minutes before each meal, was supplemented with 100 micrograms of chromium picolinate before each meal. Elevated blood lipids affected 74 percent of the study group, and 53 percent were taking prescription drugs for medical conditions related to elevated lipid levels and obesity, including diabetes medication. All the patients were taught how to alter their dietary habits and follow a sensible exercise program that included daily exercise.

The forty-two subjects who completed the study lost an average of 10.8 pounds per person. One-third of the subjects had a significant lowering of their blood lipids, including cholesterol and triglycerides levels. In eight of the cases where diabetes medication was involved, glucose levels were reduced significantly.

A recent study published in June 1998 revealed all natural weight-loss supplements provided valid results. Supplements containing HCA and chromium were given before meals with water. A nonrestricted diet regimen was used, which meant that the study subjects could continue with their usual diet.

Overall weight losses ranged from ten pounds to

twenty-six pounds during the ten-week study period. Measurement of inches lost ranged from 4.25 to 26.25 inches during the study period. All participants reported increased energy levels. The study concluded that HCA is a viable form of weight-management intervention.

With the direct relationship of diabetes and excess weight, this is yet another confirming look at the benefits of HCA as a natural supplement to improve glucose control.

Even with the many studies showing the benefits of HCA in weight reduction, glucose management, and overall sense of well-being, a large, placebo-controlled, double-blind study would be the best way scientifically to document these benefits. A study of this type is getting under way in several cities and multiple clinics across the United States. Data from this large, multicenter study are expected in mid-1999.

According to Anthony Conte, M.D., director of the LifeStyle Medical Center in Hilton Head Island, South Carolina, HCA has proven to be an excellent therapeutic approach to the treatment of obesity and weight-related disorders like type 2 diabetes. Conte has researched HCA extensively, and has published several articles using HCA as the major component in various supplements designed to help people lose weight and control their glucose levels. Conte states that during the last eight years since he completed a double-blind study on the effectiveness and safety of HCA there have been substantial medical improvements in those patients taking HCA.

The medical effects of HCA in his study include improved blood sugar levels, as needed for control of diabetes, but also decreases in cholesterol, reduction in cravings for sweets, increased lean body mass, increased fat losses, improved energy levels, and most certainly, a decrease in overall weight.

Conte has been the lead investigator in several consumer studies and has seen the same positive effects in his personal patients who see him at the LifeStyle Medical Center. Conte feels that HCA, combined with lifestyle changes, can lead to a reversal of the glucose levels in diabetic patient.

"We have noticed, aside from fat loss, an increased energy level, reduction of appetite, reduction of cravings for sweets, and a definite reduction in blood sugar levels, cholesterol, and triglycerides," says Conte. "All of these factors combined can contribute to the reversal of type 2 diabetes.

Here is a case history of one of Conte's patients who benefited within eight weeks from the HCA (containing supplemental chromium) and elements of the Diabetes Cure,

Anne Marie

Anne Marie is a pleasant middle-aged mother, fifty-one years old and only five feet, four inches tall, who weighed in at 253 pounds when she sought the help of Conte and his staff. Her excess weight had taken its toll in many ways. She had struggled with obesity nearly all her life, and had been on and off diets, trying everything under the sun to get her weight down.

Initial blood work revealed type 2 diabetes, with a blood glucose level of 172. Her cholesterol was abnormally high at 321, and her triglycerides, or blood fats, were also elevated to 276. Conte went to work, educating Anne Marie on the adverse effects of high glucose levels and the mechanisms behind the HCA, or brindle berry extract. She began to understand the interrelationship between diabetes and obesity.

Within eight weeks, she was on her way to reversing a long-standing trend. Her glucose level fell to 128 in those eight weeks of HCA use, her cholesterol had decreased to 217, and the triglycerides were down to 226. She had also lost nearly twenty pounds, and said she felt healthier as a result of being lighter.

With such clear success, she began to focus her priorities on what she needed to do to avoid a life of diabetes and obesity. She scheduled time for daily exercise. By doing that, she realized that so many of her commitments were a waste of time. She eliminated many of the "unnecessary" things she had been involved in and scheduled more time for relaxation and stress reduction.

Her status has continued to improve, mainly because she took her disease seriously.

The One-Two Punch

Although HCA alone has a powerful effect on insulin sensitivity, I add chromium to give the Diabetes Cure an added punch. Working together, HCA and chromium can increase insulin sensitivity without added side effects.

Studies examining chromium alone have shown that it:

- Increases insulin sensitivity by stimulating glucose and amino acid uptake by cells.
- Increases muscle mass in exercising humans, which is important for people with diabetes, since muscle "soaks up" and burns glucose.

- Reduces the amount of diabetes medication required when taken in combination with other diabetes medications. In an Israeli study, 47 percent of the patients who took chromium were able to reduce their levels of insulin or other medication.
- Reduces cholesterol and triglyceride levels in people with diabetes, two factors that help create complications of diabetes.

The most exciting chromium study of all was conducted by the U.S. Department of Agriculture's Nutritional Research Center. Researchers gave a total daily dose of 1,000 micrograms to a large population of type 2 diabetics in China. After four months, the group was tested and found to have blood glucose levels reduced to normal or near normal. Another group that was given 200 micrograms per day of the mineral had a significant but less dramatic benefit.

These results have led even the cautious doctors affiliated with the American Diabetes Association to say that this is a big leap.

But is it a leap in the right direction? I think it is. The combination of HCA and chromium coupled with the multidisciplinary approach outlined in the next chapter presents a powerful alternative to a drug therapy that may only forestall inevitable complications. This approach represents a holistic method of fighting this slow and silently progressive disease that does its damage with chronically elevated blood sugar.

BOX 2.1

HYDROXYCITRIC ACID AND OBESITY REGULATION

- Energy intake and expenditure is a finely regulated system in most animals.
- Body weight increases when energy expended goes down or intake goes up.
- Obesity causes greater risk for heart disease, diabetes, stroke, and other diseases.
- Obesity treatment and diabetes prevention is helped by metabolic control.
- Hydroxycitrate (-)hydroxycitric acid, or HCA, is an inhibitor of ATP-citrate lyase.
- HCA inhibits the production of enzymes that allow fat to be formed.
- HCA curbs appetite because the brain senses that caloric intake is sufficient.
- HCA causes less eating in a dose-dependent relationship in animal studies.
- The decreased appetite in those on HCA is felt to be due to metabolic processes.
- HCA was studied extensively by Hoffmann–La Roche, Inc. by A.C. Sullivan, Ph.D. and J. Triscari, Ph.D. and L. Cheng
- We must continue to seek to increase energy output and decrease caloric intake and decrease energy (fat) storage to adequately manage obesity and type 2 diabetes.

Adapted from *Appetite Regulation by Drugs and Endogenous Substances.* A.C. Sullivan, Ph.D., J. Triscari, Ph.D., and L. Cheng, Hoffmann–La Roche, Inc., Nutley, New Jersey, 139–160

My Approach

Patients don't like to work at wellness. I don't say this out of arrogance, but out of personal experience. After all, I, too, have fought my own battles with type 2 diabetes, and I know how hard it is to make changes. Nevertheless, beating type 2 diabetes calls for changes in lifestyle that aren't always easy to make. In my personal experience and in my experience with my patients, I have seen how HCA with chromium can make lifestyle changes easier.

- **HCA suppresses appetite.** Because it makes you feel full, HCA makes it easier to eat less. For many patients it eliminates even the sharpest cravings, similar to the positive effects of fen-phen and Redux.

- **HCA and chromium increase energy without giving you the jitters.** Since both medications improve the availability of glucose, you are less likely to have hypoglycemic attacks that are so common in people with diabetes. These attacks leave you exhausted and frightened, sapping you of your energy.

- **HCA and chromium battle "Syndrome X."** While HCA lowers blood fats, chromium works in tandem with it to increase insulin sensitivity. The result is a rapid change in the way you feel, because your body is getting more of the glucose that it needs, when it needs it.

These factors associated with HCA and chromium contribute to managing lifestyle changes. This is good, because the importance of diet and exercise in the war against diabetes can't be understated. I tell my patients that the fundamental thrust of treatment needs to be a multi-disciplinary approach that includes at least a new dietary regimen and daily exercise. This along with appropriate nutritional supplementation will hit the target closer than adding another medication to a long list of medications these patients are often taking every day.

I have a number of patients who have successfully adopted this approach. Below is a chart showing the improvement made by five patients who followed the Diabetes Cure. All of these patients, it should be noted, lowered their blood glucose levels to normal within four to eight weeks. This chart shows the changes in their blood cholesterol, body weight, and blood pressure brought about by the Diabetes Cure after following the program for only three months.

Initial Visit	Three Months Later
Case #1	
54-year-old female	
Body weight: 344	Body weight: 296
Blood pressure: 128/86	Blood pressure: 116/74
Total cholesterol: 174	Total cholesterol: 136
Case #2	
39-year-old female	
Body weight: 267	Body weight: 233
Blood pressure: 116/86	Blood pressure: 110/76
Total cholesterol: 265	Total cholesterol: 172
Case #3	
36-year-old female	
Body weight: 210	Body weight: 177
Blood pressure: 120/80	Blood pressure: 110/60
Total cholesterol: 260	Total cholesterol: 199

Case #4
59-year-old male

Body weight: 270	Body weight: 248
Blood pressure: 140/78	Blood pressure: 122/70
Total cholesterol: 463	Total cholesterol: 238

Case #5
62-year-old male

Body weight: 243	Body weight: 211
Blood pressure: 148/100	Blood pressure: 124/86
Total cholesterol: 252	Total cholesterol: 180

Real People

Of course, charts don't present a personal picture of the success stories that have been achieved with the Diabetes Cure. It is important to have stories as well as statistics. Several case studies of people who have followed the plan outlined in this book and the improvements they have experienced will motivate you to try the program.

Rachel: A "Quick Study"

Typical of patients on the diabetes cure is a fifty-nine year-old woman I'll call Rachel. She was determined to lose weight and control her high glucose level. She had been told several times over the years that she had borderline diabetes and as a result she would "yo-yo" diet, losing and then regaining twenty pounds over and over again.

When Rachel was tested at her annual physical examination, her cholesterol level was found to be 246, nearly 50 points above what it should have been. Her fasting blood sugar level was a whopping 230 mg/dl, well above the recommended 110. She no longer was considered borderline. This time she was diagnosed with type 2 diabetes.

Rachel decided to educate herself on her new disease. When she found that it could be reversed, she came for counseling and the alternative treatment offered through the Diabetes Cure.

She was given an HCA formulation of 1,000-milligram capsules of *Garcinia cambogia,* half of which is active substance. She was instructed to take two capsules about thirty minutes before each meal. She also kept a food diary, exercised daily, and did about twenty to thirty minutes of yoga per day to reduce stress.

When she returned for her eight-week follow-up it was clear that some things had changed. She was beaming at her eleven-pound weight loss, most of which she credited to the HCA and her food diary, which made her aware of all the snacking she did. Her cholesterol showed signs of significant improvement, too, dropping 36 points to 210. Most impressive of all was the reduction in her blood sugar level, now down to 111 mg/dl.

"I feel back in control again," she said. "I feel like I've beaten a disease that I wasn't suppose to beat."

Gary: An Engineered Approach

Another typical Diabetes Cure patient is a man I'll call Gary. He is the epitome of an engineer. Having been diagnosed at a health screening fair, he confirmed the diagnosis with a fasting blood sugar test administered by his family physician.

Knowing that most things can be fixed, he read everything he could find about the disease. With his personal computer in front of him, he designed a weekly schedule that involved eating, exercise, weight reduction, and stress control.

He was prescribed HCA tablets and chromium and instructed to take them thirty minutes before each meal. As with other patients, his capsules contained 500 milligrams of active HCA.

After eight weeks on HCA he lost almost twelve pounds and lowered his cholesterol from 180 mg/dl to 160. His blood sugar, formerly in the high 200s, was now 97.

"I just followed the instructions," said Gary, when he was praised for his health improvement. "I kept telling myself that the disease is worse than the cure. That was what convinced me to stay on track."

Bill: "I'll Do What I'm Told"

Bill, a burly sixty-two-year-old, was shocked to learn he had elevated blood sugar. It really should have come as no surprise. He loved sugar and had no dislike of fat, either. Every morning he started his day with about three cups of coffee, each cup sweetened with a couple of packets of sugar. He disliked the pink packaged sweetener and heard awful things about the blue one, so he stuck with the good old-fashioned granular, which he had done for years.

His visit to his doctor was just a routine checkup, until he was told that his weight of 314 pounds was literally killing him. His blood pressure was in the dangerous range and his blood sugar was 277 mg/dl. "It must have been the doughnuts I ate yesterday," he joked. But he knew that wasn't possible, since he hadn't had anything to eat for ten hours prior to the examination. Surprisingly, his cholesterol and triglycerides were not elevated.

Bill represents a typical older patient, somewhat set in his ways, with little insight into the dramatic effects nutrition plays on health. He had always been overweight, in the middle 200s, but lately the pounds kept coming on. In fact, when he looked back at his weight, during the last four months he had gained 16 pounds.

Bill is in the age group who usually listen to their physician. "I'll do what you tell me," he said to me when I told him about HCA and what it would take to accomplish the Diabetes Cure.

He didn't deny that he could begin to watch the sugar, the sweets, the excess fats, and he was determined to begin an exercise program. He understood the need to begin slowly to avoid hurting himself and to avoid setting too-high goals initially. He also began taking a product with HCA in it three times daily, slightly before meals. With only a few exceptions, he remembered to take the capsules.

At his eight-week follow-up, his fasting blood sugar was down to 165, while his weight had dropped to 309, and his exercise level was up to twenty minutes, five times a week. Bill felt much better, and boasted that he found he could go all week without ice cream in the evening, thanks to the HCA.

But What Will My Doctor Say?

Some people are afraid of their doctors. They see them as authority figures, inflexible and all-knowing. They think they will be rejected or ridiculed by the "white coat" if they mention a new treatment for a common disease like diabetes.

The possibility of such a response is always there, but I have noticed that even the most rigid of my peers are showing flexibility. New medical research has shown medical doctors that a minimal reliance on heavy-duty drugs is not only effective, but sometimes best. They have also seen the public embrace this holistic approach to medicine. Public polls have made it clear that people want to be actively involved in their own health, and this means trying a variety of alternative treatments.

Because of what doctors now know about holistic treatments, and because of the involvement that the public wants, my peers are more willing to help their patients try a different approach to healing. Indeed, the entire medical establishment is changing its feelings about holistic treatments.

Already, doctors are advocating lifestyle change instead of drugs as a way of avoiding type 2 diabetes. "You don't have to become diabetic if you don't want to," said Alan J. Garber, M.D., a guru of diabetes treatment. And I say that you don't have to stay one. The guidelines in this book will take you down a road toward healing. Don't try to do it alone. Even though you don't need a prescription to purchase HCA and chromium, you should not try to treat yourself without the medical professionals who make up your diabetes care team. Take this book with you and tell your doctor what you would like to do. Make sure you impress upon your doctor that you are ready to work hard to make your diabetes better.

I guarantee that a good doctor appreciates an interested and involved patient.

3

Nine Steps to a Cure

Kelsey had a lot going against her when she decided to follow the Diabetes Cure. The thirty-six-year-old secretary had a family history of diabetes, high blood pressure, heart disease, and stroke. She developed type 2 diabetes in her twenties and had progressed through the oral medications and intravenous insulin until she was now using an insulin pump to control her glucose levels. She was also taking a prescription blood pressure medication that kept her blood vessels from contracting.

The combination of diabetes, high blood pressure medication, and excessive body weight (Kelsey weighed 206 pounds at five feet, four inches) left her exhausted by the middle of the day. She began to wonder what the years ahead would be like and saw the answer to her question in her own family. Her father was nearly housebound by his own diabetes and high blood pressure, while her mother was depressed about being in the early stages of type 2 diabetes and getting worse. One of her uncles had suffered for years from diabetes and had recently had a stroke that left him partially disabled.

Not wanting her own condition to worsen, Kelsey began to follow the nine steps of the diabetes cure. "I want to become engaged again in my health care," she declared, when I asked her why she decided to pursue an alternative treatment for her diabetes.

Kelsey began a program of HCA and chromium supplementation. She also began to watch her diet very carefully, avoiding fried and fatty foods with a newfound diligence. She began to cross out times on her day planner to schedule when she was going to walk, deciding to exercise for twenty minutes before her shower in the morning and again at noon.

She followed the other parts of the nine-point program, too, including taking several vitamins as well as finding meditation time for herself to break the stress spiral.

Within eight weeks she had lost twelve pounds. More important, her cholesterol had dipped below 210 and her glucose level to 98. She has continued to stay on the program and is using much less insulin from her pump. She has now begun to talk to her endocrinologist about how she can get rid of her pump and return to, as she puts it, "an untethered life."

Her health status has improved, as those of many others have, by following the nine steps of the Diabetes Cure:

1. See your physician for a thorough consultation and examination.

2. Follow your physician's guidance and take your HCA and chromium.

3. Prepare yourself.

4. Exercise daily, actively and passively.

5. Eat a healthy diet, and don't stray.

6. Fight oxidation with vitamin supplements.

7. Stay stress-free.

8. Monitor your progress daily.

9. Pursue a positive attitude.

Although this may seem like a lot to do, this advice must be followed to foil a disease like diabetes, even if you decide to use prescription medication.

Unlike the "old days," when people took medication and did little else to fight chronic disease, more people are willing to be actively involved in treating their condition and preventing complications. A study of baby boomers diagnosed with diabetes found that they were 50 percent more likely than older patients to discuss specific ways to prevent complications. That means baby boomers are more proactive about their health. Although they become angry, frustrated, and depressed at hearing about their disease, the study says they are more likely to do something about it.

HCA and chromium are only the beginning of the Diabetes Cure. They are an important part of a nine-step program that attacks this insidious disease from all sides.

Undertaking any project, even a health project, is fun and exciting at first. When first hit with the diagnosis of diabetes, or borderline diabetes, when they are just getting into the "health of it," many of my patients are gung-ho. Reading, charting, tracking, and monitoring are actually reported to be fun. The honeymoon wears off for most of us, though, as the dreary days of winter set in, or the glucose meter runs out of strips, or we look at a cake and think, "Just one piece won't be so bad."

Diabetes, whether severe, mild, or borderline, must be carefully and intently dealt with. This is not a forgiving medical problem. This disease takes what it wants when no one is looking! Before beginning the nine steps to a cure, sit quietly for a few minutes and perform a reality check. We know a lot about the nature of this disease and how various components interact with it. This is a disease requiring great respect and perseverance, but it is a controllable disease.

The nine steps outlined in this chapter will guide you to taming diabetes. The nine steps are designed to be realistic and attainable and will work for you if you expend the effort to follow them.

Read the steps below carefully and answer truthfully, "Can I follow this step?" If you can, you will be following a path to self-improvement and healing.

Step 1: See Your Physician for a Thorough Consultation and Examination

Current guidelines from the American Diabetes Association urge all adults age forty-five and over be tested for diabetes. If the test results are normal, they should be tested again at three-year intervals. Anyone with the risk factors listed below—even children—should be tested more frequently:

- Those who are 20 percent above ideal body weight.
- Women who have given birth to babies weighing more than nine pounds.
- Anyone with parents who have had diabetes.
- People with high-risk ethnic backgrounds (African American, Hispanic, Native American, Asian).
- People with hypertension, defined by the American Diabetes Association as 140 over 90.
- People with elevated blood lipids.
- People who have previously been found to have impaired fasting glucose or impaired glucose tolerance.

BOX 3.1

PROGRESSION OF DIABETES

Factors Involved in Acquiring Diabetes

Genetic predisposition, environment, nutrition, obesity, lifestyle

Causes of Impaired Glucose Tolerance

Increase in insulin resistance
Increase in insulin levels
Transient increases in glucose levels
Increase in total cholesterol
Decrease in HDL cholesterol
Increase in triglycerides

Causes for the Onset of Diabetes

Atherosclerosis—cardiovascular disease
Elevated blood glucose levels consistently
Elevated blood pressure

Further Progression of Diabetes

Retinopathy—Eye disease
Nephropathy—Kidney disease
Neuropathy—Nerve damage

Late-Stage Complications

Blindness
Renal (kidney) failure
Coronary artery disease
Amputation
Other organ damage

If you have diabetes already, you are probably very familiar with the following tests and how to interpret their results. These tests give you a baseline from which to work, because they reveal your blood glucose levels.

Random plasma glucose test. This is the simplest way of detecting diabetes. It is usually the first test done by a doctor who suspects diabetes as the cause of symptoms like frequent urination, sudden weight loss, blurred vision, and extreme thirst. It is simply a blood test that measures the amount of glucose in your blood.

To conduct the test, a doctor will draw blood and have it tested in a glucose meter. The test relies on the fact that diabetes keeps your blood sugar levels above normal most of the time.

Results. Test results of 200 mg/dl or higher mean that you likely have diabetes.

Although this test is very effective in detecting diabetes, I prefer the following one.

Fasting plasma glucose test. This routine, cost-effective method of screening can be done by your doctor. A close version of this test can be performed at home on a glucose meter, which is available at most drugstores. Whether done at home or at the doctor's office, this test requires that you not eat food or drink anything but water for a full eight hours before taking it.

If a doctor is involved, he or she will draw blood to be tested by an in-house glucose analyzer or an independent laboratory. Your doctor will likely order other tests at the same time to get a complete profile of your blood.

If you do this test at home, you will have to calibrate the glucose meter to ensure the accuracy of the test. It is essential that you follow the directions provided with your glucose meter, because the tests are very specific. You will also have to draw your own blood with a needle stick in the finger.

Results. Test results of 110 mg/dl or under is considered normal. 110 to 125 mg/dl is considered impaired. Levels of 126 mg/dl and over indicate diabetes.

To be sure. The new criteria for diagnosing type 2 diabetes indicates that the test must be confirmed by a second reading on a different day.

Two-hour glucose tolerance test. The two-hour test is recommended by the World Health Organization and is performed by drinking 75 grams of glucose dissolved in water. Two hours later, blood is drawn and the plasma glucose concentration is measured.

The two-hour test replaced the eight-hour test, which called for an eight-hour fast followed by the glucose cocktail. Blood was then drawn six times over the next six hours. A one-hour version of this test is recommended by the American College of Obstetrics and Gynecology for pregnant women who suspect they have gestational diabetes.

Results. A nonfasting patient with a value of 200 mg/dl or greater on two separate occasions of taking the two-hour glucose tolerance test is diagnosed with diabetes.

Any of the above tests will give you a baseline from which to improve your blood glucose levels.

Step 2: Follow Your Physician's Guidance and Take Your HCA and Chromium

If you have type 2 diabetes or borderline diabetes and want to follow the Diabetes Cure, it is important to talk to your doctor about how to make the gradual switch from the pharmaceutical methods of blood glucose control you may currently be on to this more natural method.

If you have borderline diabetes or have had diabetes for only a short time, it will certainly be easier to be weaned off the diabetes drugs than if you have had the disease for a long time. Be sure to get an evaluation from a medical doctor, a doctor of osteopathy, or an endocrinologist. They will want to administer a complete physical examination and provide some biofeedback in the form of a blood test.

The test I use to monitor my patients is a fructosamine assay. This test is able to "average" your glucose levels for the past three weeks to see how consistent your blood sugar levels have been.

Another excellent test for monitoring your progress is glycohemoglobin test, or hemoglobin A1-C, which monitors glucose control during the last three months.

I prefer the fructosamine test because it allows me to look at a two-week "snapshot" of blood sugar levels and make medication or other changes faster. It also provides a shorter period between feedback, which most patients like since they want to know how well they are progressing.

I cannot emphasize enough: Do not stop or reduce your levels of medication without medical supervision.

BOX 3.2

Diagnosing Diabetes

Diagnosis	Fasting Glucose	Random Glucose
Normal	Less than 110 mg/dl	Less than 140 mg/dl
Impaired glucose tolerance (IGT)	Greater than or equal to 110 mg/dl and less than 126 mg/dl	Greater than or equal to 140 mg/dl and less than 200 mg/dl likely
Provisional diabetes (must be confirmed)	Greater than or equal to 126 mg/dl	Greater than 200 mg/dl

Criteria for diagnosis of diabetes mellitus:

- Symptoms of diabetes plus casual plasma glucose concentration greater than or equal to 200 mg/dl. Casual is defined as any time of day without regard to time since last meal.

  OR

- Fasting plasma glucose (FPG) greater than or equal to 126 mg/dl. Fasting = no food for eight hours.

  OR

- 2 hour plasma glucose greater than or equal to 200 mg/dl during an oral glucose tolerance test. Glucose tolerance challenge is using a 75-gm anhydrous glucose in water.

A thorough history and examination should be performed by your health care provider upon your request. During the initial visit, you will be asked to provide some background medical information that your doctor will review to determine if there are any risk factors for diabetes and other diseases.

This history can uncover symptoms that alert the doctor to other problems that need to be addressed for your total care. If you have diabetes, the history will help determine if there are any other problems that need attention.

You should be proactive and provide your doctor with certain information whether or not it is included on the form. This will help your physician evaluate your risk.

- Symptoms of diabetes, such as excessive urination, thirst, periods of light-headedness, or hypoglycemia.
- Prior screening test results for diabetes, such as fasting or random glucose tests.
- Prior special tests for diabetes, like oral glucose tolerance tests.
- Prior glycohemoglobin results or fructosamine tests (glyco-protein tests).
- Food intake patterns, weight history, gains or losses, diets, current nutritional status.
- Prior diabetes treatment programs or educational classes.
- Current treatment program for diabetes or weight management.
- Physical fitness level, exercise history, current exercise regimen.
- Complications of diabetes, if any; when, where, and how severe.
- Current and previous infections, especially of the skin, feet, teeth, urinary tract, and chest.

- Recurrent yeast infections or thrush (oral yeast infections) in the mouth and throat.

- Complications of diabetes of the eyes, nerves, heart, skin and feet, intestines, kidneys and bladder, sexual problems, blood vessels in the arms, legs and brain.

- Current and previous medications used to treat illnesses, both short- and long-term.

- Risk factors for heart disease like smoking, high blood pressure, obesity, high cholesterol and high triglycerides, and family history of heart disease.

- Family history of diabetes and other "hormone" diseases.

- If female, history of large deliveries (babies weighing nine pounds or more), toxemia, stillbirth, excessive amniotic fluid.

- Any other factors that may cause you to be at increased risk for diabetes or would enter into the treatment approach to diabetes, like lifestyle, culture, economic status, education, psychological issues, level of support at home, time required for self-management of this disease.

This is a long list, but one that will provide your physician with the information needed to give you the best possible care.

This assessment should be conducted yearly. If new problems arise, your doctor should be informed. Of course, if the problems are of an urgent nature, notify your doctor immediately.

Once you and your doctor review the history, the doctor will perform a physical examination. A complete physical means different things to different people, even in the medical profession. To evaluate you for diabetes, a physical examination should include the following:

- Height and weight and calculated body mass index, or BMI.
- A body composition is recommended but is not available in most offices. This test measures the amount of body *fat* (fat tissue) as compared to body *lean* (muscles and bones). The result is usually a percentage of fat.
- Sexual maturation (for children and adolescents).
- Blood pressure, pulse rate, respiratory rate, and temperature.
- Eye exam, both screening reading and with an ophthamoscope. A formal eye exam by an ophthalmologist or eye specialist is preferred so the eyes can be dilated and a detailed exam performed.
- Examination of the ears, nose, and throat, including the thyroid gland.
- Examination of the lungs, heart, and abdomen.
- Examination of the pulses in the arms, legs, and neck.
- Examination of the nervous system by touch and reflexes.
- Examination of the skin over the body, especially the hands and feet.
- Other areas may be examined based on age and gender, like the rectal, Pap smear, and breast exam for women; rectal, prostate, and testicular exam for

men. These additional tests should be performed according to national screening guidelines but can be requested by you prior to the exam.

- Various cancer screening tests may also be recommended based on your age and gender, like a mammogram for women and a sigmoidoscopy or hemoccult testing to look for colon cancer for both sexes.

The clinical examination and the history are added to a comprehensive evaluation of blood tests that are performed by a laboratory. Basic blood and urine testing will look at over fifty values of different things occurring in your body, including:

- Fasting plasma glucose levels.
- Total cholesterol.
- HDL (good) cholesterol.
- LDL (bad) cholesterol.
- Triglycerides.
- Blood chemistry, including, sodium, potassium, creatinine, blood urea, nitrogen, and others.
- Urinalysis, looking for elevated glucose, protein and ketones and infections.
- Serum albumin (protein).
- Thyroid tests and thyroid stimulating tests.

Other Tests

Other tests might include an EKG, or electrocardiogram to look at the heart and chest X-rays if you smoke. If the doctor suspects anything based on the history, other tests could be indicated as well.

The examination usually concludes with a summary from the physician on the findings of the exam. Sometimes the doctor, as I do, will ask you to come back in a few days to go over the results in detail. Since there are so much data to bring together, and the results of the tests take some time, it is usually beneficial to return for a summary visit.

After careful review of the results of your history, examination, and testing, your doctor will work with you to develop a plan for improving your health, or keeping you on the right track if you are without problems. With your baseline health established, you will now be ready to take full advantage of Step 2, which is taking the HCA and chromium supplements.

Correct Dose, Right Time

The two supplements, HCA and chromium, combine to curb your appetite, metabolize fat, and, most important, increase your sensitivity to the insulin produced by your pancreas. To achieve the maximum benefit of these supplements, you need to take the correct dosage at the proper time.

How Much Should I Take?

I recommend taking about 1,500 milligrams to 6,000 milligrams of *active* HCA per day, and about 800 to 1,000 micrograms of chromium per day. Doses should be taken three times per day, one hour before each meal, with sixteen ounces of water.

I emphasize *active* because only about half of the

garcinia contained in the supplements is actually HCA. The remainder, as with any herbal preparation, is plant matter that is not used by the body. This difference between garcinia content and active HCA has been taken into consideration in the product chart below.

Research has shown that it is virtually impossible to take too much, or "overdose," on HCA. Researchers liken its toxic effects to citric acid, the substance that gives oranges, limes, and other citrus fruits its tangy taste. If you were to take very large quantities of HCA you would certainly suffer from stomachaches or other gastric disorders, but that would likely be the extent of your discomfort.

I generally recommend that patients with delicate digestion take the lowest recommended dosage for several days before increasing the dosage to give their stomachs time to adjust to the new supplements.

Within a few days your glucose tests should reflect the effects of the HCA/chromium supplementation and the other steps in the Diabetes Cure. Most of my patients see their glucose levels rapidly approaching normal. Those who are taking medication are able to take less and less, which I recommend doing only after they talk to their physicians.

Even patients who are not able to stop taking medication entirely are able to reduce the amount they have to take. Almost all patients who follow the steps in the Diabetes Cure report more energy and vitality, and the ones who need it report a loss of weight.

The list of HCA products below represents supplements that I and other practitioners have used in the treatment of type 2 diabetes and other weight-related diseases.

The chart gives you detailed information about each product, including:

- The name and location of the manufacturer.
- The telephone number for ordering.
- The amount of active HCA contained in the tablet or capsule.
- The cost per bottle and the number of tablets or capsules contained in each bottle.
- Other supplements that are mixed with the HCA, including chromium, other minerals, vitamins, and herbs like kava and St. John's wort.

Step 3: Prepare Yourself

Making lifestyle changes is not easy, and the full effect of the Diabetes Cure cannot be attained without making changes in the way you live. Read the rest of this book and ask yourself these questions:

- Am I willing to exercise at least thirty minutes every day?
- Am I able to put stressors in second place behind my good health? Will I apply the lessons in the chapter (7) on stress control to events happening at work? Events happening at home? Emotions in my personal relationship? Bad feelings I might have about myself? Read that chapter and see if you are willing avoid stress in your life. Surprisingly, many people aren't or can't for one reason or another.
- Am I willing to watch my diet? Will I eat only "safe" foods and not cheat?
- Will I take vitamins and minerals on a daily basis?

TABLE 3.1   HCA-CONTAINING PRODUCTS

CAUTION!—Always consult your health care provider before beginning any supplements or nutritional products.

CAUTION!—Not intended for children or for use during pregnany or breastfeeding.

HCA-CHROMIUM COMBINATION PRODUCTS

Product Name	Manufacturer, Location, Phone	Garcinia /(-) HCA
Ultimate HCA	I.D.E.A. Concepts Englewood, CO 80111 1-877-311-4332	1500mg /750mg
Super HydroxyMax	HealthMax, Inc. Renton, WA 98055 1-888-469-1112 1-206-362-1111	833mg /500mg
Super CitriMax Plus	Natrol, Inc Chatsworth, CA 91311 1-800-326-1520	667mg/400mg
HydroxyMax	HealthMax, Inc. Renton, WA 98055 1-888-469-1112 1-206-362-1111	500mg /250mg
Juice Plus+ Thins Wafers	NSA, Inc. Memphis, TN 1-800-274-5830	312mg/156mg
Hydroxycitrate Plus	Metagenics Eugene, OR 1-800-338-3948	500mg/250mg
TIPTOP-PC-3	Touchstone Health Products Hilton Head, SC 1-888-984-7867	300mg/150mg
Lipodex-II	LifeStyle Medical Center Hilton Head, SC 1-843-689-2870	500mg/250mg
LITHE-3000-PLUS	LifeStyle Medical Center Hilton Head, SC 1-843-689-2870	1000mg/500mg
CITRIDYN-3	LifeStyle Medical Center Hilton Head, SC 1-843-689-2870	1000mg/500mg
CitriMax Plus*	Natrol, Inc. Chatsworth, CA 91311 1-800-326-1520	500mg/250mg

HCA-Containing Products Lists, Daily goal for HCA is 1500mg–600mg divided before meals. Chromium-Containing Product List, Daily goal 6000 for chromium is 1000 mcg divided with meals.

Cost/ Bottle†	# Caps/ Tabs	Form	Other
$39.95	90	Tablets	Highest Potency HCA–Chromium Product, Chromium 100 mcg, Vanadium (BMOV)
$63.00	90	Tablets	Chromium 100 mcg from ChromeMate* brand polynicotinate St. Johns Wort 90, Kava, 5HTP, Vanadium 150 mcg from BMOV HCA from *Super* CitriMax,* B6, Folic Acid, Ginger
$39.95	180	Tablets	Chromium 100mcg from ChromeMate* brand polynicotinate, Advantra-Z ™, Spirulina, B6, Vanadium from BMOV, Genestra HCA from *Super* CitriMax*
$35.95	90	Tablets	Chromium 75 mcg, B2, B3, B5, Manganese, L-Carnitine
$15.00	60	Wafers	Trivalent chromium 37 mcg, Lecithin, Absorbalene* Chewable Wafers (Apple Cinnamon or Chocolate Nougat)
$29.95	90	Tablets	Chromium 75 mcg, B2, B3, B5, Mangenese, L-Carnitine
$39.95	180	Capsules	Chromium 75 mcg, Creatine Monohydrate 500 mg HCA from Citrin*
$35.00	84	Caplets	Chromium 100 mcg (Ni Chrom III GTF) HCA from Citrin*
$45.00	84	Caplets	Chromium Picolinate 200 mcg HCA from Citrin*
$50.00	84	Caplets	Chromium Picolinate 200 mcg, L-Carnitine Tartrate 200 mg HCA from Citrin*
$16.95	90	Capsules	Chromium polynicotinate, 100 mcg from ChromeMate* brand polynicotinate, Uva Ursi, Cascara Sagrada, HCA from CitriMax*

TABLE 3.1 (cont'd)

Product Name	Manufacturer, Location, Phone	Garcinia /(-) HCA
HCA-C	Hervedics, Inc. Scottsdale, AZ 85260 1-800-528-3144	500mg/250mg
Nature's Diet Caps +	Douglas Laboratories Pittsburgh, PA 15205 1-800-245-4440	500mg/250mg
Nature's Diet Caps Herbs	Douglas Laboratories Pittsburgh, PA 15205 1-800-245-4440	500mg/250mg
Weight-Less	Douglas Laboratories Pittsburgh, PA 15205 1-800-245-4440	500mg/250mg

HCA PRODUCTS

Product Name	Manufacturer, Location, Phone	Garcinia /(-) HCA
*Super*HCA	Health*Max*, Inc. Renton, WA 98055 1-888-469-1112 1-206-362-1111	1400mg/840mg
Lithe-3000	LifeStyle Medical Center Hilton Head, SC 1-843-689-2870	1000mg/500mg

CHROMIUM PRODUCTS

Product Name	Manufacturer, Location, Phone	Chromium
Chromium–GTF 200	Douglas Laboratories Pittsburgh, PA 15205 1-800-245-4440	200mcg
ChromeMate*	Preventics, Inc. Scottsdale, AZ 1-800-528-3144	200mcg
Bios Life2	Rexall Showcase International Boca Raton, FL 33487 1-888-227-3925	42mcg

* *CitriMax* is a trademark and product of InterHealth Neutraceuticals, Inc.

 ChromeMate is a registered trademark and product of InterHealth Neutraceuticals, Inc.

 Citrin is a registered trademark and product of Sabinsa, Inc.

 Absorbalene is a registered trademark and product of Natural Alternatives International.

† Approximate retail cost

Cost/ Bottle†	# Caps/ Tabs	Form	Other
$35.95	90	Capsules	Chromium polynicotinate 100 mcg HCA from Citrin*
$18.00	90	Capsules	Chromium 100 mcg from ChromeMate* brand polynicotinate
$25.00	90	Capsules	Chromium 100 mcg from ChromeMate* brand polynicotinate
$36.00	90	Capsules	Chromium polynicotinate 200 mcg, L-Carnitine, B5, B6, L-Tyrosine

Cost/ Bottle†	# Caps/ Tabs	Form	Other
$28.00	90	Tablets	HCA from CitriMax* Uses *Super*HCA (60% Extract) Highest Potency HCA-Only Product
$40.00	84	Caplets	HCA from Citrin*

Cost/ Bottle†	# Caps/ Tabs	Form	Other
$6.00 $14.00	100 250	Capsules	Chromium 200 mcg ChromeMate* brand polynicotinate
$3.95 $9.95	30 90	Capsules	Chromium 200 mcg ChromeMate* brand polynicotinate
$53.95	60	Packets	Chromium from ChromeMate* brand polynicotinate. Patented special dietray fiber complex nutrient drink fortified with
$49.50		Canister	antioxidant vitamins and other dietary supplements.

- Will I take the prescribed amount of HCA/chromium and not miss?
- Will I monitor my blood and see my doctor regularly for feedback?

If the answer to any of these questions is no, then your Diabetes Cure program will be compromised. Remember, medication alone won't stop the progress of diabetes.

Step 4: Exercise Daily, Actively and Passively

Exercise is the easiest way of making your body receptive to insulin. Why this is true isn't understood, but every diabetes treatment program calls for exercise as one of its major components.

I break exercise down into active and passive categories. Active exercise involves continuous and concerted movement like walking, running, or bicycling. It used to be thought that exercise had to leave you breathless and sweating before it did any good. A number of studies have shown that any exercise, no matter how strenuous, can be beneficial. The American College of Sports Medicine recommends at least twenty minutes of exercise three times per week. I recommend thirty to sixty minutes of active exercise every day. The reason? Every day is a new day when it comes to glucose control, especially if you want to keep your levels in a narrow range. Consistent and daily exercise will help moderate your glucose levels.

Passive exercise is the calories burned from random

acts like climbing the stairs instead of taking an elevator, or parking your car at the far end of the parking lot. This is an easy way to burn extra calories and improve your glucose control.

Step 5: Eat a Healthy Diet, and Don't Stray

This is the most difficult step for most people, largely because eating is one of our most accessible and acceptable forms of pleasure. Not surprisingly, the need to change their diet is one of the greatest concerns my patients have when I tell them they have diabetes. "Does this mean I can't eat ice cream anymore?" they ask fearfully. Or, "Will I have to quit using sugar in my coffee?"

The truth is that most people with diabetes will have to change what they eat, because they probably are not eating a healthy diet to begin with. Most of my patients consume far too many fats and sugar and have gained significant amounts of weight as a result. The added weight coupled with too little activity is probably what got them to the point of developing type 2 diabetes.

The good news is that healthy eating for a person with diabetes is no different from healthy eating for a person without it. The Diabetes Cure calls for eating from a wide variety of foods, including carbohydrates, proteins, and fat. It doesn't mean you have to give up your ice cream or your sugar in your coffee, it just might mean that you will have to eat less of those foods.

There is great benefit to following the advice in this book's diet chapter. Just as there are complications to diabetes, there are complications to poor diet. Diabetes, of course, is one of those complications, but others include strokes, high blood pressure, joint problems, and lack of energy. By eating a healthy diet, you will not only help heal your diabetes but will improve your overall health as well.

The healthy eating advice in this book is aimed at:

• Helping you reach and maintain a healthy weight.
• Keeping your blood glucose within its target range.
• Finding a meal plan that you like and are willing to live with.
• Letting you know how much flexibility exists in healthy diabetes meal plan.

Following a diet plan is important for the person with type 2 diabetes. Making you miserable is not my goal in this book, especially since you are unlikely to stay on a regular diet plan you don't like. The dietary advice in the Diabetes Cure will help you select the foods you want to eat.

You will be amazed at what eating reasonably can do to for your glucose control. In fact, the acts of combining Steps 4 and 5 can be powerful medicine in and of themselves. I have a number of patients who have been able to control their high glucose using diet and exercise alone. Although it is impossible to say exactly what causes insulin sensitivity, it is clear that "Syndrome X" is closely linked to body fat and inactivity.

The chart opposite shows the blood profile of three patients who managed their glucose for three months using only diet and exercise. In addition to lower glucose levels, notice the lower cholesterol and triglycerides, too.

FASTING PLASMA GLUCOSE TESTS

	Total Cholesterol (Under 220)	Triglycerides (Desired ???)	Glucose (Under 110 mg/dl)
Patient #1			
First month	529	3,058	206
Third month	286	539	133
Patient #2			
First month	219	543	126
Third month	63	96	74
Patient #3			
First month	207	211	148
Third month	182	131	98

This chart clearly illustrates that type 2 diabetes is a form of "hoof and mouth" disease, too much food in the mouth and not enough exercise on the hooves. That is why Steps 4 and 5 are so important to the Diabetes Cure.

Step 6: Fight Oxidation with Vitamin Supplements

The only people who used to be criticized more than those who took vitamin supplements were doctors who recommended taking vitamin supplements. Recommending them for diabetes or any of its complications was almost heresy.

Now scientists can't seem to say enough about the benefits of antioxidants. For people with diabetes, they may be indispensable. Antioxidant-containing substances such as vitamins A, C, and E and alphalipoic acid may slow the development of eye, kidney, and nerve complications as well as atherosclerosis, as reported at an American Diabetes Association symposium.

Of these, vitamin E, commonly found in vegetable oils as well as wheat germ, nuts, and green leafy vegetables, is the most promising. Vitamin E appears to reduce low-density lipoprotein (LDL), so-called bad cholesterol. In a trial at the University of Texas, researchers gave healthy patients 120 times the recommended daily average of vitamin E for eight weeks. It significantly reduced LDL oxidation and other processes that contribute to atherosclerosis.

A pilot study at the University at Bugingen in Germany found alphalipoic acid, another antioxidant, cleared glucose from the blood more quickly while improving insulin sensitivity and glucose tolerance.

A Stanford University study in the June 1996 issue of the *American Journal of Clinical Nutrition* found encouraging evidence that vitamin A supplements three to five times greater than the recommended daily average may enhance the body's ability to move glucose from the blood into the cells. A fat-soluble vitamin, A is found commonly in orange fruits and vegetables, green leafy vegetables, and liver, fish liver oils, whole and fortified milk, and eggs.

The findings of recent years have changed the negative attitude medicine has toward vitamin and mineral supplements. Although we still don't know all the subtleties of supplements, it is obvious that they should be a part of a healthy antidiabetes program.

Step 7: Stay Stress-Free

Although it is doubtful that stress can cause diabetes, there is little question that it can make it worse. It does this in two ways, and one of those is mental. When we are exposed to stressful situations, many of us have a tendency to eat or drink too much food or alcohol. Many experts think we consume extra calories because they bring us comfort in these times of distress. Some people try to overcome their stressful situation by ignoring the world around them and becoming couch potatoes. And some of us do both, sitting in front of the television with a beer in one hand and chips in the other, raising our glucose levels to new highs.

Another way diabetes can be worsened by stress is through the changes in physiology it brings. Stressful situations like traffic jams cause your body to release adrenaline into your bloodstream, triggering a "fight or flight" response. This causes your body to produce more glucose than your insulin-resistant body tissue may be able to process. The results are elevated glucose levels and a tense, even frightened feeling that can last a long time.

There are many ways of avoiding stress, especially if you know the techniques to stop it before it sneaks up on you. Chapter 7, "De-Stressing for Diabetes Care," covers the best, most effective methods of staying stress-free.

Step 8: Monitor Your Progress Daily

Monitoring your progress on a daily basis is an important part of diabetes care. The goal of daily monitoring is to keep your blood glucose under tight control and as close to normal as possible.

Physicians who treat diabetes have emphasized the importance of tight glucose control for many years. Not until recently did a major study show just how important it is.

BOX 3.3

DUET™ GLUCOSE CONTROL SYSTEM

The Duet™ Glucose Control Monitor determines levels of both:

blood glucose and
glyco-protein (fructosamine)

The rapid GlucoProtein™ (fructosamine) test reveals the recent history of glucose control—the average of continuous glucose over the past 2–3 weeks.

The fructosamine level, or "glycated serum protein," measures the level of glucose that is bound to proteins (mostly albumin) in the blood. The higher the level of glucose and the longer the glucose has been elevated, the higher the fructosamine levels.

Researchers have demonstrated that elevated glyco-proteins may be the single most important risk factor associated with the complications of diabetes. It is thought that these protein-glucose complexes form irreversible structures which are thought to cause other disease processes. These structures accumulate in the skin, arteries, and kidneys and cause free radicals which lead to inflammation in these areas. Jeff Bland, Ph.D., of HealthComm, Inc., feels that these glyco-proteins cause undue oxidation in the body and lead to biological aging.

The Duet Glucose Control Monitor is useful to help diagnose and monitor the treatments of both type 1 and type 2 diabetes, and individuals who have Syndrome X. The unit could potentially help ward patients off the problems associated with diabetes such as amputation, blindness, and cardiovascular disease. Syndrome X is associated with increased biological aging, high blood pressure, osteoporosis, obesity, cancer, and heart disease.

The monitor system unit, test strips and control solution are manufactured by the LXN Corporation. Purchasing or further information may be obtained via the HealthMax website at www. healthmax.net. or by calling HealthMax at 1-206–362–1111

The Diabetes Control and Complications Trial (DCCT) followed 1,441 people with diabetes. Half of them checked their glucose levels two or three times per day. The other half tested their glucose levels four to seven times per day.

The results surprised even some of the doctors who have long been advocates of tight glucose control. They found that intensive control of glucose reduced the risk of complications resulting in eye disease by 76 percent, nerve disease by 60 percent, kidney disease by 50 percent, and cardiovascular disease by 35 percent.

Keeping tight blood glucose control means frequently monitoring your blood with a glucose meter. These devices are about the size of a pack of cards, and give readouts of your blood sugar levels in less than a minute. Based on the results, you can quickly adjust diet, exercise, or medication to keep your blood glucose levels within acceptable range.

Using a glucose meter involves sticking your finger with a lancing device to draw a drop of blood. The blood is then put on a paper test strip and inserted into the meter.

Consumer Reports magazine tested a number of glucose meters for convenience, accuracy, and consistency, and rated the top eight:

1. Glucometer Elite.
2.. Lifescan One Touch Profile.
3. Accu-Chex Advantage.
4. Lifescan One Touch Basic.
5. Accu-Chek Easy.
6. MediSense Precision O.I.D.
7. Glucometer Encore.
8. Accu-Chek III.

My personal favorite is the Duet Glucose Monitor distributed by LXN Corp. Although this monitor is much more costly than its shelf-mates, it has the ability to perform the glyco-protein test, which measures the levels of glucose control over a one- to three-week period. This allows much less individual testing, improves compliance, allows for trends in glucose levels, and can also test the standard glucose levels.

Tight Control

For the purpose of the Diabetes Cure, tight blood glucose control means keeping your blood glucose level in the narrow range suggested by the American Diabetes Association:

Fasting Levels

Normal	Less than 110 mg/dl
Acceptable	80–120 mg/dl
Needs improvement	Less than 80 and greater than 140 mg/dl

Bedtime Levels
(new in 1998 to prevent hypoglycemia during the night)

Normal	Less than 120 mg/dl
Acceptable	100–140 mg/dl
Needs improvement	Less than 100 and greater than 160

Postprandial Plasma Glucose
(taken 1.5–2 hours after eating to see how food affects glucose levels)

Normal	less than 140 mg/dl
Acceptable	less than 80 mg/dl
Needs improvement	more than 200 mg/dl

Glycohemoglobin
(test that measures the amount of glucose that sticks to red blood cells, also known as HbA1c or GHb)

••

Normal	4.0–6.0 percent
Acceptable	6.0–7.0 percent
Needs improvement	8.0 percent

••

Although daily self-monitoring of blood glucose is important for people with type 2 diabetes, especially those on medication, the number of times you test yourself varies. Research published in *Clinical Diabetes* recommends testing enough times to reach your glucose goals. For most, three times per week will be adequate; for others four to seven times per day might be called for. My recommendation is to test yourself daily in the first several weeks of the Diabetes Cure and then taper back when you have established glucose control.

I also recommend glycohemoglobin testing at three-month intervals, or better yet fructosamine testing at three- to four-week intervals. These tests assess the results of your glucose self-testing regimen and indicate whether a treatment plan is working.

Too High, Too Low

If you test yourself and find that your glucose levels are too high, you may want to lower it by increasing the amount of exercise you are doing or by eliminating some carbohydrates from your diet. See Chapter 5, "Help Through Healthy Eating," for a detailed explanation of diet's role in glucose control.

It is also possible and very common for stress to ele-

● ●

BOX 3.4

BLOOD GLUCOSE MONITORING

ALL diabetes patients should monitor their blood glucose levels.

If you are controlling your diabetes with diet or oral medications:
Check your blood glucose levels before breakfast and before dinner, at least two to three days each week.

If you are using insulin to control your diabetes:
Check your blood glucose 4 times per day—before all meals and bedtime, at least two to three days each week or more.

Less testing is needed when test values are in a consistently normal range.

More frequent testing is needed when levels are fluctuaing or elevated.

Your physician may request that you check your levels more or less frequently.

Always calibrate your glucose monitor by following the directions supplied with the unit.

● ●

vate your glucose levels. Stress can come from a number of factors, including:

- Illness.
- Infection.
- Being upset.
- Being angry.
- Being frightened.

If you think that any of these factors is leading to elevated glucose levels, see Chapter 7, "De-Stressing for Diabetes Care."

If your glucose level is too low, you should evaluate your diet. Are you eating too many simple carbohydrates? Are you eating too few calories in general? Also assess your exercise habits, since too much exercise can cause glucose levels to drop. Examine your medication intake, since taking too much can cause blood sugar to be removed from your blood at a very rapid rate.

When you feel the symptoms of hypoglycemia (moodiness, shakiness, dizziness, numbness in the arms and hands) test your blood glucose levels as soon as you can, or eat a small amount of carbohydrates to alleviate the feelings.

The American Diabetes Association recommends basing carbohydrate intake on your blood glucose levels. On the average, 5 grams of carbohydrates raises blood glucose about 15 mg/dl. Your blood glucose goal is about 120 mg/dl. Below is a chart that the association provides for raising your blood glucose levels. Note: One teaspoon of sugar equals about 10 grams of carbohydrates.

If Your Blood Glucose Is:	Eat This Much Carbohydrate:
Under 40 mg/dl	30 grams
40 to 50 mg/dl	25 grams
51 to 60 mg/dl	20 grams
61 to 80 mg/dl	15 grams
Over 80 mg/dl but have symptoms	5 to 10 grams

Step 9: Pursue a Positive Attitude

One of the greatest tonics of all is self-encouragement. To accomplish this, stay aware of your goals. Of course, this can be difficult.

There are so many pressures in life. Add to those coping with a chronic disease like type 2 diabetes, and you have an additional set of pressures most people don't have.

When pressures mount up, most of us fall back into familiar patterns of behavior because they are, well, comfortable. Many of my patients with diabetes suffer setbacks when they revert to eating (usually overeating) as they used to, or failing to exercise. Some forget to take their medication because they can't get accustomed to a new routine, or they become overly stressed about events in their lives instead of remembering that it may have been poor coping techniques that got them into the lifestyle habits leading to their diabetes to begin with.

Since diabetes is a silent disease, especially in its early stages, people often don't necessarily feel better as a result of their lifestyle changes, because they didn't really feel bad to begin with. When this happens, it is difficult to make changes. After all, they ask, if I don't feel really awful, why should I change my lifestyle anyway? Thinking like that leads many people to wait until much later in the disease process before they deal with their diabetes. The longer you wait before involving the healing process, the longer it takes to heal.

It is difficult to break the old routines and replace them with healthy new ones. New and healthy routines form the backbone of the Diabetes Cure. There isn't a pill made that will slow, stop, or reverse diabetes alone. All medications take the concerted effort of the eight steps above.

So how do you stay motivated through this treatment?

One method I recommend to my patients is to keep a daily record that includes their blood glucose count, what they eat, how much they exercise, and how they feel.

The support of family and friends will also help you stay motivated. Make sure they understand what you are trying to do by following the Diabetes Cure.

- Have family and friends read this book, so they will understand its multidisciplinary approach to fighting this disease.

- Ask them to be supportive by encouraging you toward your goals instead of away from them. This is especially true in the dietary arena, where they might try to encourage you to have one more serving of dessert or an extra helping of mashed potatoes.

- Ask them to participate in various parts of the program. Although they might not have diabetes, maybe they could benefit from a change in eating habits or an exercise program. Remind them that it is easier to make lifestyle changes if more than one person is involved.

People with diabetes have more ups and downs than the general population. Much of the depression that comes from diabetes is the realization that you have to cope with a chronic disease. It is known medical fact that people with chronic diseases have more depression than those without.

Depression is more common among people with diabetes, largely because of the physiology of the disease. I call this "blood glucose depression" because it can be brought on by variations in your glucose levels.

It is important to be aware that many times the "blues" you are experiencing can be eliminated by bringing your glucose under control. Fighting back against this depression by following these steps will help you win against these bouts of the blues and make you feel in charge of your disease.

Does the Diabetes Cure Work?

The Diabetes Cure is a unique approach to the treatment of type 2 diabetes. It offers a nonprescription medication and steps for putting you back in control of your life. At the very least, the vast majority of patients with type 2 diabetes who follow this program will show significant improvement of their disease. Of course, this program works best with borderline diabetics (people on the verge of getting the disease) and those who have not had the disease longer than five years or have not progressed to taking insulin. It does have a positive effect on virtually everyone who follows it.

Here is how the program has worked for some people.

J.R.: "So Many Things to Do"

One of our diabetic patients, J.R., is thrilled with the results of the Diabetes Cure regimen. He is a fifty-two-year-old black male with several of the common diabetes complications. In spring 1997 he decided to take a more active role in his diabetes management after a visit to our clinic.

Being a busy man, he freely admitted that focusing on his health was usually not high on his priority list. "I have so many things to do all the time and not much time to do the things that I know I should," he said. He agreed to become more involved with his disease and was very open to the learning process.

In March 1997 a screening blood sugar revealed a glucose level of 299, well over the desired range of 65–110. His liver enzymes were also elevated, and his total cholesterol showed a high level of 259. His "good" cholesterol, or HDL cholesterol, which should be at a minimum of 45 or well over, was only 42. His "bad" cholesterol was 180, higher than the recommended level of 130.

I ordered a test that would show us how well his overall diabetes control had been the last three months. The measurement of this test provides a glimpse of how long the glucose level has been high by measuring its effects on glucose binding to red blood cell components, namely hemoglobin. This is called a glyco (for glucose) hemoglobin (for the protein in a red blood cell that carries oxygen) test. The glycohemoglobin test, sometimes referred to as a hemoglobin A1-C (HbA1c), is useful in following how well our interventions against diabetes is working. Many doctors are not using this test to follow their patients, but they should be, according to the diabetes experts.

His test came back an 8.8. The normal value for the test is 4.2–6.5.

With a knowledge of how much he would have to progress, J.R. began taking the Diabetes Cure. He increased his physical activity and visited with our clinical nutritionist, Soheyla Radfar, Ph.D., who found that J.R. was eating an excessive amount of deep-fried foods, refined sugar, and red meat. He was asked to try to improve his choices each day.

Dr. Radfar taught him about the foods he was already eating and explained which ones were good for him and which ones weren't. Suggestions were made to alter the way the food was prepared to keep the flavor and get rid of fat.

Things began to change in J.R.'s life. He began to lose weight, to drink much more water than before, and to eat smaller meals four to five times a day. He didn't feel hungry.

He was walking ten to fifteen minutes, four to five times a week, and was changing his daily routine to fit in more exercise. His wife even joined him on several of the walks when she could. The walks helped him "unwind" from his hectic day and pay attention to his body. Now he trimmed the fat off his meat and ate a piece of fruit on the way home from work instead of stopping for a milkshake. He was changing his lifestyle, and it wasn't as hard as he thought it would be.

When he came in for his checkup, J.R. was pleased to see that his blood pressure had dropped. The results of his blood test showed a man who had changed for the better. His glucose level was now 105, well within normal, his glycohemoglobin test, which was previously 8.8, was now 7.1—not normal but quite improved. His total cholesterol level was down to 192, while his LDL or bad cholesterol was down to 135, and his risk factor for heart disease had dropped considerably. J.R. was pleased indeed.

J.R. continued to follow the suggestions for the Diabetes Cure, and his glycohemoglobin level was found to be 5.4 only four months after he began to focus on his health.

Sean: "I Feel Better"

Sean is a fifty-seven-year-old man with non-Hodgkin's lymphoma that has been complicated by hypertension and diabetes for years. His blood glucose levels were always elevated, sometimes very high. He had a difficult time emotionally with the daily fluctuations and felt as if nothing he did could control the varied results. He was discouraged with these fluctuating numbers and at time felt, "What's the use, no matter what I do, I keep getting bad results."

Diabetes can be very discouraging for many people who react like Sean. They try to become involved in their disease but the feedback they get keeps telling them that, no matter what they do, the glucose numbers will still be off.

Sean had begun searching for an alternative approach to help him with his diabetes when he found our clinic. He appreciated the traditional medical approach to his cancer, but wanted to help this traditional approach by including alternative treatments for his diabetes. He heard a lecture I gave at a local natural health food store on the values of HCA for those interested in controlling their diabetes in a natural fashion, and was intrigued by what he heard.

He was seen by our clinical nutritionist, who explained the pros and cons of HCA. After that, he was determined to begin using the fruit extract. He was given two tablets three times daily of a form of HCA that contained 500 milligrams of garcinia, yielding 250 milligrams of active HCA. The formulation also contained 75 micrograms of chromium. In addition to the HCA and chromium, the supplement contained vitamins B2 (riboflavin), B3 (niacinamide), B5 (pantothenic acid), manganese, and L-carnitine.

By his report, within just the first two weeks, he began to "feel better." When questioned in detail about what this meant to him, he stated his energy level was improving, his eyesight was improving, and his glucose had fallen an average of 10 points on routine testing.

He increased his exercise, which he was now able to do with his renewed energy levels. He has continued to improve by using the HCA/chromium compound and compliance with the other steps in the Diabetes Cure.

Sean's case points to the fact that often diabetes does not stand alone as a single disorder. Type 2 diabetes frequently comes along with a variety of disease states and can actually be missed altogether by an untrained eye or by the health care provider who is focused on the presenting problem only. High sugar levels, as seen with type 2 diabetes, can slow healing and interfere with recovery of a variety of conditions. A problem with glucose handling should always be in the back of the minds of patients and their physicians.

Mike: "Full-Blown" Trouble

A patient named Mike illustrates a classic case of full-blown type 2 diabetes out of control. Presenting to our office with a blood sugar of 351 mg/dl, Mike decided to face his problem head-on.

"I never really thought about it much," he said. "I just kinda tried to watch my sugars sometimes. If I didn't feel bad, I thought I was okay."

This is such a typical, yet unfortunate, error in a patient's perception of his disease. Diabetes doesn't knock on the door and announce itself with symptoms as so many other diseases do. Diabetes waxes and wanes, causing trouble undetected. Mike realized that testing was the only way he could tell if his values were high.

My nutritionist instructed him in the essentials of a good diet for diabetics and what food choices would push his blood sugar levels up. She described the actions of HCA and chromium and the benefits of these compounds.

Mike declared that he was determined to focus more on his health and devote at least thirty minutes a day to active exercise, something he had never done.

His focused energy paid off. Four weeks later, we all rejoiced at his progress. His glucose fell to 190 mg/dl, down from his initial of 351 mg/dl, his exercise was consistent, and his food choices were dramatically improved. Best of all, he felt great!

Mike has "learned to live better" through the Diabetes Cure and has continued to improve by following the steps of the program.

These are just three patients who have been helped by the Diabetes Cure. Results are seen anywhere from four weeks to three months, depending on the severity of the disease and how well the patient complies with all the steps. Although HCA and chromium have both been shown to work independent of the program, they are far more effective when used in conjunction with all the other steps.

Megan: "I Just Want to Avoid It"

Megan is a sixty-year-old patient who wants no part of "getting old."

"I don't have time for it," she says with a devilish grin. "I want to do everything as natural as possible, not that I have anything against the prescription stuff, I just want to avoid it if I can."

Megan said she was an only child who usually didn't take "no" well. When she was diagnosed with type 2 diabetes and told she had "no" choice but to go on medication, she decided to come to me to see what kind of natural regimen she could follow.

Our nutrition staff went to work, outlining her daily recommended exercise requirements, the foods she should eat more of and the foods she should avoid. She took detailed notes.

She was given HydroxyMax, a combination of HCA and chromium, two tablets, three times daily, before meals.

Megan liked her new "glucose control project" and saw it as one she could master, "no sweat."

We recommended an EKG, blood testing, and an exercise treadmill test before the start of her exercise regimen in addition to the recommended physical examination.

She passed with flying colors and couldn't wait to get started on her walking program. We insisted that she stay on the recommended slow-start program, as she had not been exercising routinely. She agreed, and within two weeks was up to walking a half hour per day.

Retesting of her blood after two weeks revealed a fasting blood glucose level of 110 mg/dl, well within the normal range and nearly 100 points lower than when she started. Her six-pound weight loss at the end of a month was testimony to her dedicated spirit and rapid change in lifestyle, for the better.

Megan is a good illustration of my sixty-plus-year-old age group. Frequently they will embrace the elements of the Diabetes Cure very well, because it gives them something to do!

Many retired or "winding down" sixty-year-olds are finding themselves with little idea about what to do after retirement, and they become bored. Some become intimately involved with the daily soap operas, and pass their lives from episode to episode. Many others find a renewed joy in becoming healthy.

It is this age group that is at most risk for developing the "silent diabetes" of type 2 diabetes mellitus. As Megan tells her friends, "Don't be afraid of finding out you have type 2 diabetes, be afraid of NOT finding out you have it!"

Nine Steps to Better Health

There you have it, the nine-step Diabetes Cure. Although it won't put an unconditional end to type 2 diabetes in some people, it will at least reduce the amount of prescription medication that has to be taken to keep your glucose levels under control and to keep the devastating complications of diabetes at bay.

The Diabetes Cure requires more time to take hold than prescription medicine because it is a holistic approach. You can expect to see changes in the amount of prescription medication you are taking in about two to four weeks. Even though HCA and chromium alone will most likely have positive effects on your blood glucose levels, the Diabetes Cure works best when all of the nine steps are followed.

4

Exercise That Fights Diabetes

The Program

How much? At least thirty to sixty minutes of continuous exercise *of any type.* This is recommended by the Centers for Disease Control and the American College of Sports Medicine. *How often?* Every day, with no excuses.

Why? Any exercise reduces your risk of getting diabetes and increases your sensitivity to insulin if you do have diabetes. A substantial amount of research that proves this. Vigorous exercises (running, hiking, bicycling) have for a long time been shown to improve insulin sensitivity. More recent research has shown that nonvigorous activity like walking and even household chores can have a very positive impact on diabetes.

The value of exercise in controlling and avoiding type 2 diabetes has been made obvious to me a number of times by the effect it has on patients. One such patients was a man named Ed, a fifty-five-year-old biology teacher with a growing spare tire around his middle and a worsening glucose problem. Tests showed him to have high glucose levels, and his physical symptoms—dizziness, sudden exhaustion, excessive urination—indicated that this silent disease was beginning to get noisy.

Believing that less medication is most often best, I tried a novel approach: an exercise prescription. I explained that for some reason, exercise helps the muscles "suck up" glucose and use it. If he could walk regularly—for at least thirty minutes per day—and eat no more than he was eating, I speculated he would need no other form of intervention.

Ed liked the idea and followed this simple exercise prescription religiously. Every morning he got up an hour earlier and walked for more than thirty minutes. Nothing stopped him. If it rained, he wore a rain suit. If he slept through the alarm, he walked at lunch or in the evening. For one month, he walked diligently. His symptoms disappeared and his glucose levels dropped into the safety zone.

For Ed, exercise alone was the solution to his diabetes problem. For you, it might be different. There is always one truth: Exercise, along with healthy eating, is one of the most important things you can do to keep your blood glucose levels in check and to minimize complications from diabetes. That's because exercise usually lowers blood sugar and helps your body use the food you eat in a more efficient way.

At the same time, exercise appears to help insulin work better. That important information was reinforced recently by the University of South Carolina. In studying a racially mixed group of nearly 1,500 participants, researchers found activities ranging from sports and vigorous exercise to hobbies, household chores, and even sleep all had a positive effect on insulin sensitivity. Reduced insulin sensitivity is one of the risk factors for diabetes as well as for heart disease.

If you're overweight, exercise, along with careful attention to nutrition and medication, can help take off extra pounds. Losing those extra pounds can help reduce the need for medication and minimize diabetes complications. There are more reasons that exercise should be an important part of your diabetes treatment plan. They include:

Benefits to the cardiovascular system. Regular exercise, especially aerobic exercise—the kind that makes you sweat and your heart beat faster—improves the way your heart, lungs, and blood vessels work. It decreases overall blood cholesterol and increases the levels of high-density lipoprotein (HDL), so-called good cholesterol. When ten marathoners were checked after they ran a race, their HDL had gone up as much as 10 percent. One study from Brigham and Women's Hospital in Boston found men with diabetes who exercised strenuously at least once a week saw their risk of heart attack plummet 50 percent compared with those who didn't exercise at all. More frequent exercise reduced the heart attack risk further.

High blood pressure control. Exercise can help bring down high blood pressure, which is associated with stroke and heart attack. One study involving Harvard University alumni found those who were active had a 20–40 percent lower chance of having high blood pressure.

Studies also have shown that those who exercise regularly have a slower resting heart rate; their heart also beats more slowly when they're exercising than the hearts of people who are out of shape. A slower heartbeat and lower blood pressure translate into good news for those who want to stay healthy. Both have been shown to slow hardening of the arteries or even to reverse it.

Glucose control. Exercise helps remove glucose from your body. So if you have type 2 diabetes, exercise may help you control your blood glucose with little or no medication. This occurs because exercise improves glucose transport and insulin sensitivity, reducing insulin resistance for eight to forty-eight hours after exercising. Work with your health care team to develop your personalized exercise program. Remember, never alter the amount of diabetes medication you take without approval of your physician.

Increased muscle strength and flexibility. Strength-building exercise increases the muscle-to-fat ratio. When combined with stretching, the result can be a body that's stronger, has greater muscle tone, and bends and flexes more easily. Weight-bearing exercise, such as working out with weight machines or free weights, or just walking, is especially important for women because, in combination with a healthy diet, it can preserve bone mass and reduce the risk of osteoporosis.

There is also a mind-body connection to physical activity that can lift your mood. First, physical activity distracts you with an enjoyable activity that takes the immediate focus off your disease. Second, exercise increases the release of endorphins, according to a study at the University of Wisconsin, Madison. These naturally occurring brain chemicals affect how you feel. Exercise raises body temperature, which may result in brain chemical changes that help ease anxiety. Either way, exercise is especially important for people with diabetes, who may experience depression as a natural part of their disease.

Weight loss. Carrying extra pounds reduces your body's sensitivity to insulin. Losing weight and keeping it in a normal range helps your body make more efficient use of the insulin it produces and may lower the risk of diabetic complications.

Improved body image. How you look is directly related to how you feel. Being physically fit improves muscle tone and circulation, and can help control body weight while also helping you remain active and able to participate fully in your own life and in the care of your diabetes.

The overall benefits of all types of regular exercise for everyone, not just people with diabetes, increasingly are being recognized. Even after genetic disorders and other risk factors are considered, people who exercise regularly are much less likely to die prematurely than their sedentary counterparts, Finnish researchers report. Those who vigorously walk or jog for an average of thirty minutes six or more times a month, considered "conditioning exercisers," had a 43 percent lower risk of death than sedentary people, according to the study of about 8,000 sets of twins.

Even people who were occasionally active had a 29 percent reduced risk of dying compared to more sedentary people, says Dr. Urho M. Kujala, an expert in sports and exercise medicine at the University of Helsinki. In the study, published in the *Journal of the American Medical Association*, Kujala and colleagues observed similar risk reductions when they looked specifically at individual twin pairs in which only one twin was active. This suggests risk factors that run in families may be overcome, in part, with exercising.

Ralph Paffenbarger, M.D., of Stanford University, in his research on the physical activity of 17,000 Harvard alumni, discovered those who were more active lived longer. Death rates came down steadily as the subjects burned off more and more energy by doing such things as stair climbing and walking. He noted that people who took part in rigorous sports had the lowest death rates, but not far behind were people who pushed themselves to some degree but not so hard that they broke out in a sweat. How much does a person add with exercising? According to Paffenbarger, every hour working out boosts the life span by an hour. It's almost like free time.

Start with Your Doctor

A talk with your doctor is absolutely essential before beginning any exercise program. In addition to assessing your overall physical health, your doctor can determine the kinds of exercise that are right for you. This decision should take into account certain kinds of exercise you should avoid if you have diabetic complications such as degeneration of the eye known as retinopathy, heart disease, or kidney and nerve damage.

People with diabetes have a different physiologic reaction to exercise than people who don't. During aerobic exercise, those without diabetes generally have no change in blood glucose levels because the liver responds as demand for glucose increases.

Those who have diabetes generally experience a decrease in blood glucose no matter what their preexercise level of blood glucose. People with diabetes should talk in detail with their health care teams about how to recognize the symptoms and avoid hypoglycemia.

Practice Random Acts of Exercise

Despite the many benefits to being physically fit and active, more than 60 percent of U.S. adults don't get the recommended amount of activity they need; 25 percent aren't active at all, according to a 1995 Surgeon General's report. A busy schedule at home and at work, inclement weather, boredom with the current exercise program, occasional illness, and inertia can lead even the most dedicated person to slack off and eventually give up.

But there is good news. All exercise counts. According to a 1995 issue of the *Journal of the American Medical Association*, the accumulation of thirty minutes or more of moderate-intensity physical activity every day can pay off in enhanced health. The guidelines were based on studies developed by researchers from the Centers for Disease Control and Prevention and the American College of Sports Medicine. Such light workouts can even relieve anxiety, Indiana University researchers have found.

Called "random exercise," it can be a great way to extend or add to your regular exercise program, but take note—the operative word here is *accumulated*. If you're dedicated, creative, and motivated, you can get the exercise you need, improve your overall health (including blood glucose levels), feel better, and maybe even live a longer, healthier life. Remember that the next time you're tempted to circle a parking lot a second time looking for a parking spot near the door.

Indeed, the benefits of random exercise can and do make a difference in your good health and to the reduction of your diabetes complications. Some possibilities include:

- **Yard work**. Mowing your own grass, raking leaves, weeding or using a broom instead of a leaf blower are all good fitness sources. When done vigorously, they have the added benefit of aerobic exercise that also increases strength and flexibility. Other possibilities—car washing, gardening, mulching flower beds, and gutter cleaning.

- **In the house**. Vacuum carpets and scrub floors, wash windows and clean out closets. Not only will you gain in fitness, you'll feel generally better about your living environment. Other possibilities— washing baseboards, waxing the floor, making beds, shaking rugs, painting a room, and hanging clothes on the line.

- **At work**. Instead of calling someone on the next floor or in the next building, walk over. Use a portion of your lunch hour or break time to walk in the halls or around the building. Be sure to swing your arms and walk briskly to gain maximum benefit. Other possibilities: Pausing every hour to leave your desk, do lateral stretches and twists, move your arms, and touch your toes.

- **Just for fun**. Skip the golf cart and carry your own clubs on the course. Bypass dessert and go for a walk after dinner. With your doctor's approval, pick up a light-intensity fitness activity that has a social component, such as walking at the mall, bowling, dancing, or skating.

- **Around town**. Instead of driving, walk from store to store. Carry your own groceries to the car. Facing a long delay at the doctor's office? Spend the time walking briskly in the halls. Other possibilities: Walk in the park, volunteer as a playground supervisor at a local school, or take a water aerobics, weight lifting, or yoga class.

Focus on Fitness

Random exercise is a way of augmenting a regular exercise program, but it won't meet all your body's needs for strength, aerobic, and flexibility exercise. To develop a well-rounded exercise program, talk with your health care team about your lifestyle, exercise preferences, overall health, and diabetes management. Work together to figure out ways to make a complete fitness plan a normal part of your life, one that fits in naturally and also meets your needs. It should include:

- **Your fitness preferences**. If you hate team sports or running, find alternatives.
- **Balance and variety**. Doing the same activity every day is boring and could mean you're overworking one muscle group to the detriment of another. Vary your program by walking one day, taking a dance class on another day, and cutting the grass with a push mower on another.
- **Your schedule**. A night owl who signs up for an early

morning aerobics class is destined for failure. By creating an exercise program that fits with your personal style, you're more likely to persist.

- **Willingness to seize opportunities**. Park your stationary bicycle or ski machine in front of the television and work out while watching the evening news. At work, walk to the rest room at the opposite end of your floor. Don't saunter in the grocery store, walk briskly. It will save you money and, in combination with carrying your own groceries, build strength.

Enjoyable exercise is the kind that falls naturally into the rhythm of your day. If your fitness activities feel dull or pointless, it's time for a change. Even though rigorous workouts normally are better for the body, most of the good results of exercise can be had through any form of activity that pushes the body somewhat.

How hard should a workout be? The answer to that question is very individual and should be based on your total health. The American College of Sports Medicine says it's best to exercise at 60 to 90 percent of your maximum heart rate. Though, again, any activity is better than no activity. Harder activity tends to strengthen the heart more and to be better for the body in general.

You can chart a proper workout level by subtracting your age from 220. That number is your maximum heart rate, in terms of beats per minute. Then the number should be multiplied by .60 to find the lower end of the "target" workout range and .90 to find the higher end of the range.

For instance, if you're forty, subtract your age from 220 to get your maximum heart rate—180 beats per minute. Multiply this figure by .60 and .90. That gives you your target range; in this case a pulse rate of 108 to 162 beats each minute. Here are target heart workout rates for normal people of various ages:

TARGET HEART RATES

Age	Target Range Beats Per Minute
25	117–175
30	114–171
35	111–166
40	108–162
45	105–157
50	102–153
55	99–148
60	96–144
65	93–139
70	90–135
75	87–130
80	84–126

To measure your heart rate during a workout, stop exercising briefly and puts two fingers on your neck just below your ear or on your wrist. Simply count the number of beats in ten seconds and multiply that number by six to come up with the heart rate for one minute.

Exercise Safety Guidelines

People with diabetes face special challenges when it comes to staying fit. To make the most of your fitness program:

- Know your blood glucose level before, during, and after exercise.

- Keep a quick source of carbohydrates with you at all times—for example, a nondiet soft drink, dried fruit, or glucose gel or tablets.

- Get an exercise buddy. If you must exercise alone, tell others where you are going and when you'll be back.

- Begin every workout with a warm-up and end it with a cool-down.

- Drink plenty of water before, during, and after your workout.

- Carry diabetes identification. If possible, also carry a cellular phone and/or money for a phone call.

- In very hot or cold weather, exercise indoors— consider walking at the mall or purchasing exercise equipment for your home.

Nix Nicotine

You know that smoking is bad for your cardiovascular system, but did you know that for a person with diabetes, it's even more urgent to quit? Here are the facts. According to a new study, British epidemiologists at University College in London followed 4,427 people with diabetes for fourteen years. Compared with people with diabetes who had never smoked, those who had quit more than ten years ago still had a risk of death from all causes that was 25 percent higher. Those who had quit more recently had a death risk 53 percent higher. The researchers speculate smoking plus diabetes multiplies damage to the heart and blood vessels, accounting for the unusually high risk among ex-smokers who have diabetes.

Quitting smoking reduced death risk compared with current smokers, but risks remain unusually high for diabetic ex-smokers. And it's not just *your* smoke that can affect your health. Exposure to secondhand smoke is worst for those with diabetes as well as those with high blood pressure, a new study shows. Researchers defined "exposure" to secondhand smoke as spending at least one hour a week near at least one smoker.

People exposed to secondhand smoke are at greater risk for atherosclerosis, the buildup of artery-narrowing plaques. In a study of 10,914 middle-aged adults, researchers found those who were exposed experienced a 20 percent increase in atherosclerosis progression compared with those free of secondhand smoke exposure. Atherosclerosis in the people with diabetes who were exposed to secondhand smoke progressed even faster.

As a person with diabetes, you know the risks of life-threatening complications from your disease are high, so take action. With so many options to choose from when it comes to giving up your nicotine addiction—support groups, nicotine replacement systems, and behavior modification—you've never had a better time to quit. Talk with your health care team about the best way for you to manage your nicotine addiction and reduce the increased risk of diabetic complications that smoking presents.

Preventing Hypoglycemia

The risk of hypoglycemia keeps many people with diabetes on the sidelines. With careful management and the help of your health care team, you can learn to exercise while also managing your disease. Here are the basics:

- Plan to exercise one to three hours after a meal, when blood glucose is rising or peaking.

- Monitor your blood glucose levels, and if necessary, snack before or during exercise. How much you should snack depends on your overall health, your ability to control your blood glucose levels, and the type of exercise you're doing. For instance, if you're biking, walking, or golfing, a high-carbohydrate snack such as six ounces of juice or half a plain bagel should do the trick. On the other hand, if you're doing intense exercise such as aerobics, running, or racquetball, half a meat sandwich with a cup of low-fat milk is called for.

- Know the symptoms of hypoglycemia and respond promptly with an fast-acting sugar source such nondiet soda or fruit juice, raisins, hard candy, or glucose tablets.

- Know how your body responds to particular kinds of exercise by checking your blood glucose levels before, during, and after exercise.

If you feel a hypoglycemic reaction coming on, stop immediately and have half a cup of orange juice, a nondiet soft drink, or three glucose tablets.

Athletes and other very physically fit people may have a lower risk of hypoglycemia because their conditioning allows them to better store glucose in their muscles. These same people may be at higher risk for postexercise, late-onset hypoglycemia. This condition may occur up to twenty-four hours after exercise and is more likely after a sudden increase in training load or a long or high-intensity workout. The best way to prevent this type of hypoglycemia is awareness, plus careful meal planning and adjustment of insulin during and after exercise. If you believe you fall in this category, talk with your health care team. They may suggest you meet with an exercise physiologist or other health care professional familiar with the care of athletes who have diabetes.

Exercise in a Perfect World

An intense workout should include three basic parts:

- A five- to ten-minute warm-up with gentle stretching. As you warm up, avoid bouncing, as it can injure muscles that aren't fully ready to work.

- Twenty to thirty minutes of aerobic activity that raises your heart level, but doesn't cause straining or shortness of breath. As a good rule of thumb for the aerobic part of your program, you should be able to exercise and carry on a conversation. Can't do it? Slow down a bit until you can talk comfortably.

- Five to ten minutes of cool-down exercises, stretching, or slow-paced walking.

A good exercise program should make you feel better, not worse. It's true, you may be a little sore the next day, but don't let minor muscle stiffness stop you. Just invest a little more time in your warm-up to stretch out those newly challenged muscles and begin again.

If you haven't exercised in a while or have been ill, you may find you can do only five to ten minutes of aerobic exercise before you begin to strain. Listen to your body and slow down. Do what you can and return to your exercise program the next day. By gradually increasing the length and intensity of your workout, you reduce the chances of injury and increase the chances that you'll stick with it.

The good news about aerobic exercise is that the benefits don't stop when you do. Your body continues to burn calories at a higher rate after your workout. The number varies, depending on the intensity of the workout, your overall fitness level, and your muscle mass. Since muscle burns many more calories than fat, the benefits can increase as your strength and muscle mass increase.

Exactly how often you should and can exercise depends on many factors, including:

- Your overall health.
- Blood glucose levels and control.
- Your lifestyle.
- Any diabetes complications.

In general, schedule some type of fitness activities daily. You may want to alternate days when you do aerobic exercise with days when you do strength-building or flexibility-enhancing activities. Or you may want to keep the same consistent program. The most important thing is, with your physician's approval, get active and stay active.

Warning

For people with diabetes, sometimes exercise isn't a good idea. Talk with your doctor about your specific medical history and don't exercise if you:

- Are ill or recovering from an illness.

- Have diabetes that has affected your nerves (called neuropathy) or your eyesight (retinopathy), and haven't discussed with your doctor the impact of exercise on these complications.

- Are following your care plan, but continue to have difficulty keeping your blood glucose levels under control.

- Have a blister or open sore on your foot.

- Haven't checked your blood glucose levels.

- Haven't eaten.

- Haven't talked with your health care team to develop a fitness strategy.

Foot Facts

Peripheral nerve damage can lead to a loss of sensation in the feet. This loss of sensation may mean a blister goes unnoticed and becomes infected. For the person with diabetes, that infection can be deadly. Diabetic complications is the fourth leading cause of limb amputation. Make attentive foot care an integral part of your fitness program.

- Buy fitness shoes that fit well. The shoe should have plenty of room in the toe box, fit snugly at the heel, and feel absolutely comfortable from the start. Shop for shoes in the afternoon when your foot size tends to be largest and try them on wearing your workout socks. Spending the extra time and money necessary to get a shoe that fits perfectly is a long-term investment in your feet.

- Break in new shoes slowly by wearing them for an hour or so, then switching to another pair.

- Change shoes every day and allow them to air and dry out between wearings.

- Wear clean socks that are a combination of cotton and polyester that wick moisture away from your feet at every workout. You may consider purchasing socks with extra cushion and arch support for exercise or any time you expect to do a lot of walking.

- Inspect your feet daily for blisters, scratches, redness, or tenderness, and talk with your health care team if you find any of these.

- Never walk barefoot, not even indoors.

- Wash your feet daily and dry between the toes carefully. If your physician recommends it, apply lotion, but avoid getting it in between the toes.

- Trim your toenails with the contour of your toes. Talk with your health care team if ingrown nails are a problem.

Weight a Minute

Exercise melts body fat. Even though people who work out tend to eat more than couch potatoes, exercisers tend to have less body fat. Less fat means less of a load on the heart and circulatory system, and less fat means that you need less insulin. So how does a person reap the benefits of exercise and push life to its limits without undue strain? It's not all that hard. Plenty of exercise can be gotten with tiny lifestyle changes. And the process can actually be fun.

Average Calories Burned in Exercise Per Minute

Knowing the value in calories of some of the common forms of exercise can help motivate you. It also can be especially important if you're trying to get fit while also losing weight. The number of calories you burn varies with the intensity of your workout and with your size. Here are some exercise options and calorie-burning ranges per minute of exercise.

ACTIVITY	WEIGHT IN POUNDS			
	105–115	127–137	160–170	182–192
Bicycling, indoor	11	13	15	17
Skiing cross-country, moderately hilly terrain	9	11	18	16
Running	9	10	12	13
Step aerobics	9	10	14	17
Jumping rope, 100 skips per minute	9	11	15	17
Volleyball	8	9	11	12
Handball	8	9	11	12
Basketball	7	8	10	11
Stair climbing	6	7	8	9
Aerobics	6	7	8	9
Hiking, 4 miles per hour, 20-pound pack	6	7	8	9
Tennis, doubles	6	6	8	8
Square dancing	6	6	8	8
Cross-country skiing, ski machine, 11 miles per hour	6	6	8	10

ACTIVITY	WEIGHT IN POUNDS			
	105–115	127–137	160–170	182–192
Treadmill, 13.5 miles per hour	6	6	8	10
Downhill skiing	5	7	8	9
Gardening	5	6	7	8
Roller-skating	5	5	7	7
Calisthenics	4	5	7	8
Weight training, moderate resistance	5	6	7	8
Skating	5	5	6	7
Walking, 15 minutes per mile	5	6	8	9
Swimming	4	5	5	6
Sexual intercourse	4	5	5	6
Rowing	4	5	5	6
Walking, 20 minutes per mile	4	4	6	7
Golf	3	4	4	5
Bowling	3	3	5	5

Wellness Walking

When it comes to a fitness payoff, nothing beats walking. It's free. When done at an appropriate level of intensity, it's usually injury- and pain-free. Best of all, walking is a normal part of most people's day. To gain maximum fitness benefits from it, all you have to do is more.

Start small—five to ten minutes a day is a good way to begin, especially if you haven't exercised in a long time or you're newly diagnosed with diabetes. By starting with a short increment, you can build up stamina and strength, plus the confidence you need to exercise often and well, despite your diabetes.

Walk at a pace that's invigorating and enjoyable. Move your arms briskly and inhale and exhale deeply to gain maximum benefit. Increase the length and speed of your walk slowly to allow your body to adjust and adapt. If you feel pain or strain, return to your most recent level of activity and start anew.

If goals motivate you, work over a period of weeks and months to a level of four miles per hour. If goals are a disincentive for you, just work toward gradually increasing the duration of your walks.

On the Run

Some people would rather run than walk. And it can be a great workout if you're properly warmed up, wearing appropriate shoes, and accustomed to the increased demand it places on your body. Running or jogging can be hard on your joints and feet. For people with diabetes who are already at risk for foot injuries, that can be a concern.

If you've talked to your doctor and gotten the okay to hit the jogging path, start by using a walking/running approach. Begin by warming up your muscles, especially those in your legs, and walking briskly. Once you feel warmed up, move to a jogging pace, and continue until you feel winded. Then fall back to a brisk walk until you've recovered your breath, then return to jogging. Over time, you'll probably be able to jog the entire distance of your chosen route. At that point, you may want to alternate jogging days with walking days.

Where you run is up to you, but it's best to avoid

cement, which is especially punishing on the joints. Consider a local track, paths in your neighborhood park, or the grass along the sidewalk. Remember to listen to your body and slow down if you experience breathlessness or pain, especially in the joints.

Walker/Jogger Safety

- Wear shoes that are comfortable and allow your feet to breathe.
- When working out outdoors, dress appropriately for the weather.
- Always walk or jog facing traffic.
- If walking at night or near dusk, wear light-colored clothing and a deflector vest, and carry a flashlight.
- Wear your diabetes identification and be sure to tell someone where you're going and when you expect to be back.

Strength Training

Building muscle as a part of your exercise program has many benefits. Strong muscles help you cope with everyday activities, whether you're carrying groceries, toting your luggage on a business trip, or working in your yard. Strength training is a way you can work to prevent broken bones due to osteoporosis. An extra advantage to weight training is that well-toned and larger muscles burn more calories.

According to a study from the American College of Sports Medicine, weight training may lower total cholesterol by 4 percent. More important, it may lower low-density lipoproteins (LDL), so-called bad cholesterol, by as much as 13 percent while boosting HDL by as much as 5 percent. This cholesterol-lowering benefit is especially important for people with diabetes, who are at a higher risk for cardiovascular disease.

Strength training usually involves repeated lifting of hand weights and/or the use of weight machines. As your strength increases, the number of lifting repetitions and the weight of the items being lifted are increased. There are many approaches to this activity. If endurance is your goal, lift moderately heavy weights fifteen to twenty times, rest, then repeat. If strength plus endurance are your goals, use a weight you can lift only eight to twelve times and rest between sets.

Talk with your health care team about which approach is right for you. You may be referred to an exercise physiologist who can assist you in determining the best approach, proper lifting techniques, and appropriate weight for you to begin with.

Many people do strength training at fitness clubs where they have access to a variety of strength-building machines and the supervision of trainers or other professionals. You can gain many of the same benefits with hand weights at home. You can even create your own hand weights by filling quart or half-gallon soda bottles with measured amounts of sand or water.

Smart Weight Training

Before beginning a weight-training program, talk with your doctor. This can be especially important for people with diabetes, since weight training can, in some cases, worsen diabetic complications such as retinopathy. Other safety first weight-training strategies include:

- Start with five to ten minutes of aerobic exercise, such as walking, running, or calisthenics to warm muscles.

- Breathe in when lowering weights and breathe out when lifting weights.

- Work out with a buddy or a trainer who can watch for problems in your technique, spot you when you're using heavy weights, and provide encouragement.

- Either alternate your weight-training day with a rest day when you focus on flexibility and endurance activities, or work muscles in the upper body on one day and the lower body the next.

- Cool down after your workout by walking, stretching, or doing a slow-paced stint on a stationary bike or ski machine.

Staying Motivated

If you keep doing what you're doing, you'll keep getting what you're getting. That's good news when it comes to a fitness program. Unfortunately, motivation can wane, and your well-planned schedule can get interrupted. Suddenly a week has gone by and you've not so much as laced up your athletic shoes. Here are some tips to keep your exercise plan on track:

- **Do it often.** One way or another, everybody should work out at least three times a week. That schedule allows a day off in between exercise days to let muscle soreness go away. But this is a minimum. With a gradual buildup, it's safe to work out four or five days a week, or even every day.

- **Do it long enough.** Exercise sessions should be at least twenty to thirty minutes. But that's a minimum. Anyone who exercises more than this does his or her body more good.

- **Set goals that work for you.** Begin gradually and increase the intensity and duration of your workout over time.

- **Harder isn't necessarily better.** Perhaps you've heard, "No pain, no gain." That couldn't be further from the truth. Pushing yourself to a level where you feel pain can result in injury and more than a little reluctance to continue working out. Instead, focus on the time spent exercising, not on making the exercise hard. Constancy and consistency are the keys.

- **Spice it up.** Variety is the spice of exercise life. Shift the kinds of fitness activities you do with the seasons or with your family and work schedule. Above all, make your fitness fit your day, not the other way around.

- **Get a buddy.** A buddy can help keep you motivated and give you someone to compare your progress with.

- **Map your personal progress.** Track how well you've improved with a workout diary. Tracking your success, along with the success of your diabetes management, is one way to keep motivated.

- **Reward yourself.** Have you reached a milestone goal? Have you been especially diligent in sticking with your fitness and overall diabetes management plan? Reward yourself with a new pair of workout shoes, a class that teaches you a new fitness skill, or a change in your exercise routine that makes it easier for you to maintain your commitment.

Exercise and Pregnancy

Whether you developed gestational diabetes as a part of your pregnancy or were living with type 2 diabetes before you became pregnant, exercise plays an important part in your good health. Staying physically fit throughout your pregnancy helps moderate weight gain and increases your strength and stamina.

Contrary to prevailing beliefs, exercise may lower blood sugar during gestational diabetes, if properly supervised. Experts at the third International Workshop-Conference on Gestational Diabetes Mellitus said exercise—along with a proper diet and supplements such as vitamin B6 and chromium—may help lower blood sugar. This, in turn, may reduce health risks to mothers and fetuses.

Monitoring your blood glucose levels is especially important during pregnancy, because the level can drop quickly as a result of exercise. Talk with your health care team about learning to maintain tight control during your pregnancy. It may mean checking your blood glucose levels seven or more times a day, but it is an investment in your continuing good health and that of your baby.

Talk with your health care team about developing a prenatal diabetes management and fitness plan. And remember:

- If you haven't been exercising before your pregnancy, this isn't the time to start training for a marathon. Instead, go for low intensity; start slowly with walking and simple, relaxed stretching.

- Follow the exercise and blood glucose testing regime your health care team recommends.
- Bypass activities that require you to lie on your back after the fourth month of pregnancy, involve holding your breath, require straining, or include jerky movements or quick changes of direction.
- Your blood sugar can drop quickly and unexpectedly during exercise, so be attentive to early symptoms of hypoglycemia. If they occur, stop immediately and have fruit juice, nondiet soda, or three glucose tablets.
- Drink plenty of liquids before, during, and after you exercise.
- Start with warm-up and cool-down stretches and limit the intense portion of your program to no more than fifteen minutes.
- Check your heart rate frequently and keep it below 140 beats per minute.
- Be aware of your body temperature and keep it below 100 degrees. Don't use a hot tub or steam bath without your doctor's permission.
- Stop exercising if you feel light-headed, weak, or breathless.
- Ask your obstetrician to show you how to feel your uterus for contractions during exercise. Contractions can be a sign that you're overdoing.

Until recently, experts thought exercise endangered the mother's health, fetal development, or both. Experts now say the only pregnant women with diabetes who should avoid exercise are those with:

- Pregnancy-induced hypertension.
- Three or more spontaneous abortions.
- Cervical incompetence.
- Fetal distress.
- Placenta previa or other placental problems.

Soothing to the Soul

Exercise is an essential part of the Diabetes Cure, but unpleasantness isn't. Feel free to try a number of different exercise activities until you find the ones that suit you best. There is more than one way to burn a calorie, and the ways you choose should be soothing to the soul as well as helpful for the body.

5

Help Through Healthy Eating

The Program

What? Develop a healthy diet that is probably different from the one you currently follow.

Why? Some doctors call type 2 diabetes "hoof and mouth disease," because it is caused by not enough hoof (exercise) and too much mouth (food). Weight gain is thought to be the primary cause of type 2 diabetes. The diet recommended in these pages controls glucose levels. It also promotes a feeling of fullness. These two factors—glucose control and feeling full—will help control or prevent type 2 diabetes. They will also help you to lose weight if you need to.

How? I recommend a diet in which 50 to 60 percent of calories come from complex carbohydrates (whole grains and high-fiber fruits and vegetables), 10 to 20 percent comes from protein (beans, fish, poultry, eggs, and very little red meat), and 20 to 30 percent from fat, with most of that coming from monounsaturated fats like olive oil.

And don't forget to watch your salt intake.

What you eat, when you eat, and how much you eat directly affect your blood glucose levels. It's as simple as that. Most people never really give serious consideration to the types of foods they eat until they're diagnosed with diabetes. Having diabetes isn't the end of your relationship with the foods you like. Instead, it can be the beginning of a healthier relationship with food and with your body.

In truth, your meal plan is ideal for anybody who wants to eat in a healthful, nutritious way. Your diet includes a wide variety of foods from all parts of the Food Pyramid, including new foods as well as the old favorites you love. When you follow a recommended meal plan, you minimize the risk of diabetes complications like heart disease, high blood pressure, and the risk of amputation or blindness, and you give your body the nutrition it needs to function at its best.

The Diabetes Control and Complications Trial, a ten-year study of the connection between closely managed glucose levels and diabetes complications, found that people with diabetes can reduce their chances of complications, but never entirely eliminate them. That's a fact that should motivate you to do all you can to manage your disease carefully.

Do you have an individualized meal plan? Most people find it helpful to meet with a registered dietitian experienced in diabetes care. Think you don't need one? Think again. Your diabetes is with you for life, so we're not talking about some prepackaged diet program that you'll follow for a few weeks or months, then return to your old eating habits. Instead, a registered dietitian will work with you to create a customized plan that determines your:

- Daily calorie intake.
- Daily carbohydrate intake in grams that will allow you to keep your blood glucose levels within your target range.

- Daily fat gram intake to keep you at less than 30 percent of calories.

- Options for breakfast, lunch, dinner, and snacks.

- Techniques for distributing your calories throughout the day so your body always has the food it needs.

- Choices for adjusting your meals (or medications) for exercise and travel.

BOX 5.1

DIABETES TREATMENT GOALS

Biochemical Parameter	Normal	Goal	Action
Post prandial glucose (mg/dl)	Less than 140	Less than 180	Less than 80 or greater than 140
Preprandial glucose (mg/dl)	Less than 110	80–120	Less than 80 or greater than 140
Bedtime Glucose (mg/dl)	Less than 120	100–140	less than 100 or greater than 160
Hemoglobin A1c (%)	Less than 6	7	Greater than 8

These values are for nonpregnant individuals. Adjust glycohemoglobin values to correspond with local differences in laboratory methods. Adapted from the ADA Standards of Medical Care for Patients with Diabetes Mellitus, *Diabetes Care* 20, Number 7, July 1997.

Ultimately your meal plan is designed to teach you an eating style that's flexible and takes into account your:

- Favorite foods and foods you avoid.
- Lifestyle, including work schedule, family commitments, and exercise.
- Target blood glucose levels.
- Ideal weight.
- Need to minimize risks of diabetes complications as well as other health risks.

Anatomy of Food

Food is fuel. The right balance of foods containing needed carbohydrates, protein, and fat, plus vitamins, minerals and micronutrients, will help your body function more smoothly. Scrimp on the quality or quantity of fuel and your body pays the price. It's true for everyone, but especially true if you have diabetes. That's because the carbohydrates, protein, and fat provide calories for energy and affect blood glucose levels.

No single food group provides all the nutrients and calories a healthy body needs to run smoothly, fight off infection, and rebuild itself daily. That's one of the reasons the Food Pyramid is an ideal tool. When you eat from all parts of the pyramid in the recommended proportions and combinations, you provide your body with an edge in maximizing good health and minimizing diabetes complications.

The fact is, all foods provide the body energy in the form of calories. Food not used immediately is stored as fat.

The challenge for most people, but especially those with diabetes, is to strike a balance between the number of calories you take in and the number you burn. That's because being overweight, even by a small amount, makes it more difficult to keep your blood glucose levels in a normal range as well as manage health-related issues such as cholesterol and triglyceride levels.

For some people with diabetes, weight management can be tricky. As they gain greater control over blood glucose levels, they may find their weight goes up. That's because, in part, they are no longer losing calories in their urine. To maintain their weight, they have to cut the number of calories they were losing before. Talk with your health care team about a weight-management program that will prevent weight gain, but reduce the likelihood of low blood sugar reactions.

Here's where using the Food Pyramid and a meal plan comes in. At the very top are fats, oils, and sweets. These should be eaten sparingly by anyone concerned about good health and keeping weight down. Next are dairy and meat/protein. Small amounts of both of these are necessary, but remember that they're higher in calories than foods at the bottom of the pyramid. You should target getting the bulk of your nutrition from the last categories— vegetables, fruit and bread, cereal, rice and pasta. These are good choices because they're major sources of fiber, vitamins and minerals, and energy that's easily accessible to the body.

Carbohydrates

Carbohydrates are your body's primary energy source. They contain 4 calories per gram, and 100 percent of carbohydrates are metabolized into glucose. Carbohydrates have a protein-sparing effect by supplying the energy needs of the body and enabling the body to use protein for growth and repair. When broken down, carbohydrates become glucose, a simple sugar that is your body's main energy source.

Complex carbohydrates are found in some vegetables, grains, cereals, and breads, while simple sugars are found in fruits, some vegetables, and milk. Simple sugars also show up in candy, soda, and other sweet treats. To maximize good nutrition, go for complex carbohydrates. They contain fiber and provide more vitamins, minerals, and dietary fiber per calorie than simple sugar. Be wary of such processed foods as white bread. Refining removes much of the nutritive value. Opt, instead, for whole grains. In general, get 50 to 60 percent of your total calories from carbohydrates.

Despite what you may have heard, how quickly glucose gets into your body depends not only on the type of carbohydrates you've eaten, but on several factors, including:

- Amount eaten.
- How foods are cooked or prepared
- Other foods eaten at the same time.

That's true even though simple sugar and complex carbohydrates are digested at the same rate, because their overall digestion may be slowed by fat present in the food.

Proteins

Proteins are used by the body for tissue growth and repair. Like carbohydrates, they provide 4 calories per gram. Even though protein is an important part of a balanced diet, don't go overboard. Unless you choose very lean cuts of meat or eat a vegetarian diet, many sources of protein can be high in fat calories.

Protein sources include meat, fish, poultry, and dairy products. When eaten in combination, additional protein sources include rice, beans, eggs, and grains. As a group, proteins provide your body with essential amino acids. Plan to get 10 to 20 percent of your total calories from protein sources.

Here are some ideas for eating your favorite kinds of meat, but cutting back on fat:

- It's all in the cooking. Skip the frying pan and grill, roast, steam, or poach meat.

- Spray away. Use a cooking spray or nonstick cookware to prevent sticking during the cooking process.

- Fixate on fin and fowl. Overall, seafood and skinless poultry are lower in fat than red meat, so make steaks and chops an occasional treat and focus on seafood and poultry.

- Go lean. Select lean cuts of meat. If tenderness is a concern, pound it or create all-natural tenderizers using citrus juices and spices.

- Be size-wise. Cut back on your portion to about three ounces. That's a serving about the size of a deck of cards.

- Go Oriental. Cook as Asians do, using very small amounts of finely sliced or chopped meat as flavoring to complement generous servings of vegetables. Then stir-fry in a nonstick pan using a nonstick spray or a tiny amount of monounsaturated oil.

- Skim and trim. Trim excess fat from meat. Chill soups, prepared broth, and casseroles and skim off fat that rises to the top.

Fats

Fat has gotten a bad reputation in the last few years. The fact is, fats are necessary in limited quantities, because they provide the fatty acids that are necessary for life. Fats are stored and used as energy reserves. The real issue is how much and which types of fat you eat.

In his *Report on Nutrition and Health*, Surgeon General C. Everett Koop took aim squarely at American's high consumption of foods laden with fat and cholesterol as two elements that make a major contribution to the high incidence of heart disease and other cardiovascular ailments in Americans. That's because excess calories from any source are stored as body fat, and unfortunately for most people, the fat storage capacity of the human body is unlimited.

Fats provide 9 calories per gram, making them the most concentrated calorie source. To make the most of good nutrition, limit your fat intake to 30 percent of your total calories. That's a good idea for everyone, but especially important for people with diabetes. If you have diabetes you are at increased risk for premature atherosclerotic vascular disease, and that can increase your risk of heart attack and stroke.

There's also a connection between the amount of body fat you have and insulin resistance. Having too much fat, especially on the upper part of your body, makes it difficult for your body to use insulin. Being overweight puts a strain on your pancreas which in turn, makes it harder for the pancreas to make the insulin you need.

Cholesterol is the type of fat most often associated with diabetic complications. Usually your body makes this substance on its own. It's essential in the making and repair of cell membranes and plays a role in the manufacture of such essential hormones as estrogen and testosterone, but it is one of the main culprits in clogging arteries and causing heart disease.

Saturated fat is found in animal and some vegetable products. To avoid these, you have to be a smart shopper and read food labels and the ingredients of foods you buy. Saturated fats show up most often in fast foods and such processed foods as commercial baked goods, cake mixes, cookies, crackers, coffee creamers, and snack foods. Even some oat bran cereals that gained popularity for their ability to lower cholesterol contain large amounts of saturated fat. While these foods may contain no cholesterol, they do contain substances such as palm kernel oil, which has been shown to raise cholesterol.

From saturated fat, the liver produces a cholesterol-rich bile that digests fat. Since saturated fats are such complex molecules, more bile has to be produced to digest them than is needed for unsaturated fat. The result? Much of the extra cholesterol ends up circulating in your bloodstream as saturated fat.

And there's more. Saturated fat reduces the number of low-density lipoprotein (so-called good cholesterol) receptors in the liver. These receptors pull LDL cholesterol from the bloodstream. If they aren't there to perform that function, the LDL continues to build.

Believe it or not, there are some fats that, when eaten sparingly, are good for you. These include polyunsaturated fats and monounsaturated fats, both of which contain fewer hydrogen atoms and don't stay in your bloodstream the way their saturated cousins do. Unsaturated fats require less bile to digest. They also bind with cholesterol and pass into the intestines into the bloodstream. In the *Archives of Internal Medicine*, Dr. Grace Goldsmith published results showing an unsaturated fat diet leads to as much as 25 percent more bile being eliminated from the body than in a saturated-fat diet. The result? Lower cholesterol levels in the bloodstream.

The ultimate goal is to get no more than 30 percent of your total calories from fat, with 10 percent coming from saturated fats.

A Word of Caution

Remember that "fat-free" on the label does not mean calorie-free, or that you can eat all you want. For instance, one ounce of real sour cream has 62 calories and 6 grams of fat, while the reduced calorie version has 45 calories and 2 grams of fat. Many fat-free cookies make up for the absent fat content by increasing the sugar. The only way to be sure of exactly how much fat and how many calories you're getting is to read the label carefully. Recommended serving size should get equal attention. Eating just two low-fat cookies can save you calories and fat grams. But some people are seduced by the low-fat label and may eat twice as many of the low-fat version, ultimately consuming more calories than if they'd eaten the regular version.

Fat Cutters

Interested in cutting back on fat, but not sure how to begin? Here are some basic changes you can make that will help you cut back on fat:

- Cut fat in recipes by reducing the amount you add. If a dish calls for four tablespoons of oil, add two and make up the rest with water. When using oils choose corn, safflower, or other polyunsaturated fat.

- Use skim milk instead of whole or 2 percent milk.

- Replace sour cream with plain, low-fat yogurt.

- Use only egg whites or egg substitutes in cooking.

- Substitute fat-free frozen yogurt, sherbet, or sorbet for ice cream.

- Substitute a fat-free artificial topping for whipped cream.

- Select low-fat or fat-free margarine instead of butter. In particular, look for margarines that have vegetable oil as the first ingredient, not partially hydrogenated oil.

- Opt for lower-fat cheese such as mozzarella made with part-skim milk, ricotta, Sapsago, and low-fat cottage cheese.

- Create your own lunch meats using skinless baked chicken or turkey.

- Select fat-free mayonnaise over traditional or homemade mayo.

The Skinny on Fats and Oils

Common Sources of Saturated Fats

- Butter.
- Lard.
- Meat fat.
- Palm oil.
- Coca butter (chocolate).
- Solid shortening.
- Cream cheese.
- Bacon and bacon grease.
- Sour cream.

Common Sources of Polyunsaturated Fats (Healthier Fat Choices)

- Corn oil.
- Cottonseed oil.
- Sunflower oil.
- Safflower oil.
- Soybean oil.
- Mayonnaise.
- Salad dressings.
- Margarine.

Common Sources of Monounsaturated Fats (Healthiest Fats)

- Olive oil.
- Canola oil.
- Avocadoes.
- Peanut butter.
- Nuts.

Fat Replacements

Fat replacements are grouped according to their source—carbohydrate, protein, or fat. Some are calorie-free replacements, others are reduced-calorie. It can be tricky to spot some fat replacements when you look at the ingredients list on a package or can. That's because many of them have innocuous names like maltodextrins, modified food starch, xanthan gum, and microcrystalline cellulose, to name a few.

Simplesse is a protein-based fat replacement made from all-natural protein derived from either egg or milk protein. Its manufacturing process gives it the smooth, tongue-coating consistency most people associate with products high in fat. The body digests and absorbs it just like protein.

Since Simplesse breaks down when it's heated, it's best suited for foods such as Simple Pleasures, an ice cream substitute with 1 gram of fat and 120 calories for a four-ounce serving. (Premium ice cream has 19 grams of fat and 276 calories per four-ounce serving.) Those figures make Simplesse look like the answer to an ice cream lover's fantasy, but only if the ice cream lover sticks to the four-ounce serving, not a double-dip cone.

Olestra is a calorie-free fat replacement made from a combination of oils and sugar. During processing, these substances form a molecule the body's digestive enzymes can't break down, nor can it be absorbed, so it passes through the body undigested.

Such snack foods as chips made with Olestra have begun to appear on the market; a cooking oil is reported to be in the works. Though Olestra can be used interchangeably in cooking with other fats and oils, some people get diarrhea after eating large quantities of food prepared with it. Most snacks prepared with Olestra are fortified with fat-soluble vitamins A, D, E, and K, because these vitamins may also be eliminated along with the undigested Olestra.

Friendly Fiber

Fiber is the indigestible portion of plant food that passes through the intestines nearly intact. There are two main types of fiber—soluble and insoluble. Water-soluble fiber slows the rate of nutrient absorption from the stomach and intestines and may be helpful in lowering blood sugar and cholesterol levels. Examples include oat bran, fruits, vegetables, beans, peas, nuts, and seeds. Insoluble fibers speed the passage of food through the digestive system. They increase the bulk of the stool, aiding in the prevention or treatment of constipation, which can be a problem for some people with diabetes. Examples include whole grains and wheat bran.

The average American diet contains only about 10 to 20 grams of dietary fiber per day. If you have diabetes, it's a good idea to work toward gradually increasing your fiber intake to 25 to 50 grams per day. Increasing the fiber in the diet too rapidly may result in excess gas, cramping, bloating, and diarrhea. Adequate fluid intake—six to eight eight-ounce glasses per day—is also important when fiber is increased.

Salt Is Everywhere

Sodium—salt—is everywhere, and the average American eats 5,000 milligrams per day. That's not hard to imagine when you consider just one teaspoon of salt contains 2,000 milligrams of sodium.

If you have diabetes, cutting back on sodium is a long-term investment in your good health. People with diabetes are at an increased risk for high blood pressure. The general recommendation for sodium intake is 1,100–3,000 milligrams per day. Hypertensive patients should restrict sodium to 2,000 milligrams per day or lower, as ordered by their physicians.

Sodium causes your fat cells to retain fluid, expanding them to as much as eight times their size. This additional weight, sometimes called water weight, is an extra burden on your body, especially your heart. Some evidence suggests that too much salt over a long time can lead to kidney malfunction, which forces the blood pressure higher.

High blood pressure and even salt itself has been shown to speed the development of atherosclerosis. Not only does the increased pressure contribute to plaque deposits, but it causes smooth muscle cells in the arteries to contract and become stiff and enlarged. The larger the artery muscles become, the smaller the lumen, the area for blood to flow through them. Taking in less sodium smoothes these muscles cells, causing them to relax to a smaller size, so the lumen area is larger.

Outside your kitchen and without a lot of label reading, it can be difficult to identify foods high in sodium, which can appear in the most unlikely places. For instance, a McDonald's milkshake has a higher sodium content than a Quarter Pounder. Sodium is even found in products such as Alka-Seltzer, sugar-free soft drinks, and penicillin. Other likely suspects include:

- Salad dressings.
- Cold cuts and processed meats.

- Canned soups and vegetables.
- Fast food.
- Some cheeses.
- Snack foods such as chips and crackers.

To reduce sodium intake, stop using salt in cooking and at the table, and avoid processed foods. Concerned that food won't taste as appetizing? Experiment with combining fresh and dried herbs and spices or adding a dash of herbed vinegar or fresh citrus juice. Other salt-reducing tips include:

- Avoid processed foods.
- Use salt substitutes.
- Eat more fruit.

Easy to Eat Sweet

Sugar substitute possibilities are everywhere. The pink stuff, the blue stuff—whatever your choice, they can help people with diabetes satisfy their sweet tooth without falling off the food-plan wagon.

Technically, most sweeteners are classified as nutritive or nonnutritive. The Food and Drug Administration (FDA) determines acceptable daily intakes (ADI) for approved low-calorie sweeteners. The ADI is defined as the amount the FDA determines to be safe to consume on a daily basis over a person's lifetime without adverse effects. It usually includes a hundred-fold safety factor. All of the following sweeteners are approved for use by persons with diabetes.

Nutritive Sweeteners

- **Fructose.** Fructose, found in fruit and honey, is one of the most common naturally occurring sugars. It is not associated with rapid or high levels of blood sugar in well-controlled diabetes. It is one to one and a half times as sweet as real sugar and contains the same number of calories. Products sweetened with fructose should be calculated into the diet as carbohydrate calories (either starch or fruit) if more than 20 calories are used at one time.

- **Sugar alcohols.** Sugar alcohols include sorbitol, mannitol, and xylitol. They contain 4 calories per gram, and they are absorbed slowly and metabolized like fructose. If you have enough insulin, the fructose will be stored as glycogen in the liver. If there is not enough insulin, the fructose can cause a rise in plasma glucose. Sugar alcohols can cause diarrhea.

- **Aspartame.** Best known as Nutrasweet and Equal, aspartame is a combination of two amino acids— aspartic acid and phenylalanine. Aspartame is 180 times sweeter than sucrose, so only a small amount is needed to get the sweetness you want. It contains 4 calories per gram but does not affect glycemia.

Nonnutritive Sweeteners

- **Saccharin.** The body doesn't metabolize saccharin, which is 300 times sweeter than sucrose. The kidneys excrete it unchanged, so it has zero calories. Although some studies have shown saccharin causes bladder cancer in animals, it's considered safe at human levels of consumption.

Smart Shopper

Feel baffled by all the food claims you see in ads and on food packaging? You are not alone. Most consumers ignore these claims or guess at their true meaning. Let your diabetes motivate you to sharpen your food-shopping techniques. Once you and your dietitian have set daily goals for calories, fat, saturated fat, cholesterol, and carbohydrates, as well as fiber and sodium, use food label information to help you shop smart. Reading food labels can be time-consuming, but it's worth it.

Start by looking at the Nutrition Facts panel that is a part of the packaging of nearly all foods sold in the United States. It tells you the basics, such as the serving size, the number of calories per serving, and the calories from fat. Serving size, in particular, deserves your attention. Many foods such as candy or snacks may appear to have modest amounts of fat and calories until you learn that only a tiny amount is calculated as a serving size.

Next comes the actual number of calories, grams of fat, cholesterol, sodium, carbohydrate, and protein in a single serving, and the percent of daily value. The percent daily value reveals the total daily intake you use with one serving, assuming you are eating 2,000 calories each day. The actual percentages may be higher or lower depending on how many calories are in your diet.

Health Claims

Food manufacturers can only make health claims on food labels that are supported by scientific research. Some of these include the relationship between:

- Calcium and osteoporosis.

- Fiber-containing grain products and cancer.

- Fruits and vegetables and cancer.

- Fruits, vegetables, and grain products that contain fiber—particularly soluble fiber—and the risk of coronary heart disease.

- Fat and cancer.

- Saturated fat and cholesterol and coronary artery disease.

- Sodium and hypertension.

- Folate and neural tube defects.

Other Claims

Manufacturers also make claims about the nutritional value of products that can be confusing. Here are some of those claims and what they really mean:

- Calorie-free. Has fewer than 5 calories per serving or other designated amount.

- Low-calorie. Has 40 calories or fewer per serving.

- Light or lite. Has one-third fewer calories than or half the fat of the foods it is being compared with, usually the full-calorie version of the same food.

- Less and reduced fat or sugar. Is at least 25 percent lower in calories or other ingredients compared to the full-calorie or nonreduced version.

- Cholesterol-free. Contain less than 2 milligrams of cholesterol and 2 grams or less of saturated fat per serving.

- Low-cholesterol. Contains 20 milligrams or less of cholesterol and 2 grams or less of saturated fat per serving.

- Low-fat. Must have 3 grams or less of fat per serving to fall in this category. This can be confusing because although vegetable oils contain no cholesterol, they are 100 percent fat. Vegetable oils are still preferable to butter or lard because they have less saturated fat. A tablespoon of vegetable oil still has about 14 grams of fat and the same 126 calories found in butter or lard.

- Fat-free. Describes a food with less than 0.5 gram of fat per serving.

- Low saturated fat. Describes a food with 1 gram or less of saturated fat per serving and not more than 15 percent of its calories from saturated fat.

- Low-sodium. Contains 140 milligrams or less of sodium per serving and per 100 grams of food. Remember sodium is also found in monosodium glutamate (MSG), sodium bicarbonate (baking soda), and sodium nitrate and occurs naturally in some foods.

- Very low-sodium. Contains 35 milligrams or less of sodium per serving and per 100 grams of food.

- Sodium-free or salt-free. Has less than 5 milligrams of sodium per serving.

- Light in salt. Has 50 percent less sodium than the regular version.

- Sugar-free. Has less than 0.5 gram of sugar per serving.

More Terms to Know

Be aware that "dietetic" has no standard meaning and only indicates something has been changed or replaced. It could contain less sugar, less salt, less fat, or less cholesterol than the regular version of the same product. "Natural" also has no specific meaning except for meat and poultry products, in which case it means no chemical preservatives, hormones, or similar substances have been added. On other food labels, "natural" is not restricted to any particular meaning by government regulation. "Fresh" can only be used to describe raw food that has not been frozen, heat-processed, or preserved in some other way.

At the Store

When shopping, aim for foods rich in vitamins, minerals, and fiber, and low in fat and cholesterol. Read the ingredients list on all food labels. Ingredients that make up the larger percentage of the product are listed first, and those that make up a smaller percentage of the total are listed last. Here are some general food-buying guidelines:

- Bread. Look for low-fat varieties with whole grains as the first label ingredient. A Swedish study has shown that sourdough bread may be a good choice. That's because its fermentation process is less likely than other breads to trigger sharp rises in blood sugar.

- Cereal. Pick cereals listing whole grains first on the label and containing 3 or more grams of dietary fiber, 1 gram or less of fat per serving, and 5 grams or less of sugar per serving.

- Crackers/snacks. Again, let whole grains be your guide and look for those with 2 grams or less of fat per serving. Try to keep the sodium content under 400 milligrams per serving.

- Rice, pasta, and whole grains. Choose converted, brown, or wild rice of any type. Look for unfilled fresh or dried pasta, preferably made with whole-grain flours. Avoid pastas containing eggs and fat.

- Frozen desserts. Choose ones with 3 grams or less of fat per four-ounce serving, especially low-fat frozen yogurt, or low-fat or nonfat ice cream. Frozen fruit juice bars with fewer than 70 calories per bar are another option. Avoid those made with cream of coconut, coconut milk, or coconut oil, which are high in saturated fat.

- Milk. Choose skim or 1 percent milk, buttermilk made from skim milk, and low-fat and nonfat yogurt that is artificially sweetened. Also consider acidophilus milk as an aid to digestion.

- Cheese. Look for skim-milk and reduced-fat cheeses with 6 grams of fat per ounce or less.

- Red meat. Choose lower fat grades of meat such as select and lean body parts, such as beef round or sirloin, pork tenderloin, and leg of lamb.

- Luncheon meat. Look for lean or 95 percent fat-free meats with 30 to 55 calories per ounce and 3 grams of fat or less per ounce.

- Poultry. Breast meat is the leanest. Removing the skin before cooking cuts fat by 50 to 73 percent and cholesterol by 12 percent. Beware of turkey or chicken luncheon meat, hot dogs, and bacon, as they can be high in fat.

- Seafood. Fresh seafood is low in fat when it's broiled, grilled, or poached, not fried. Choose canned fish packed in water or with the oil rinsed off. Look for low-sodium products.

- Vegetables. Opt for fresh and frozen vegetables, which are the most nutritious per bite. Drain and rinse canned vegetables to reduce sodium.

- Fruit/fruit juice. Choose fresh, frozen, or dried fruit, preferably without added sugar. Look for 100 percent pure fruit juice.

- Margarine/oil. Choose brands containing 1 gram or less of saturated fat per serving (usually one tablespoon).

- Soup. Choose low-sodium and/or reduced-fat varieties. For cream soups, use nonfat or low-fat milk or water in preparation.

Away from Home

Whether eating out is a special treat or a routine part of your day, keep the following in mind.

- Call ahead. Before eating in a new restaurant call in advance to ask about menu options so you can plan your food for the day.

- Ask questions. Not sure what's in a particular dish or how it's prepared? Ask questions. If the waiter can't answer, then ask for a manager.

- Develop a good eye. Restaurant portions can sometimes be huge. Help yourself by cultivating an eye for portions that fit your meal plan. Some restaurants allow you to order smaller portions at reduced prices. If larger portions are served, put the extra in a to-go box before you begin to eat.

- Go light. Ask that no butter or salt be used in preparing your meal.

- On the side, please. Request that sauces, gravy, salad dressings, sour cream, and butter be served on the side or left off altogether. Although this may seem like deprivation, try it for two weeks and you will see that restaurants frequently overload food with fatty items.

- Choose your method. Opt for broiled, baked, poached, or grilled meats and fish rather than fried. If food is breaded, peel off the outer coating to get rid of the extra fat.

- Ask for substitutions. Most restaurants will allow you to substitute low-fat cottage cheese, baked potato, or vegetables for French fries.

I recommend eating salad with low-fat dressing with lunch and dinner, since lettuce is both filling and a good source of fiber.

Last Call

Having diabetes doesn't mean you have to give up having an occasional beer, mixed drink, or glass of wine, but it does mean you'll have to plan alcohol in your diet.

Alcohol provides more calories than carbohydrates or protein (7 calories per gram), but no essential nutrients. Alcohol is broken down at a constant rate in the liver by specific enzymes, and your body burns about one ounce of alcohol per hour. Metabolizing alcohol does not require insulin, but it can cause a high or a low blood sugar, depending on the circumstances surrounding its use.

Consumed with a meal, it has a tendency to add calories and possibly increase the blood glucose. On an empty stomach, it can cause significant hypoglycemia in patients on insulin. That's because the alcohol inhibits gluconeogenesis, the formation of sugar from protein and other sources. The hypoglycemic effect may persist for as long as twelve hours after the last drink.

To be on the safe side, use alcohol in moderation. The symptoms of alcohol intoxication and hypoglycemia are similar, so it's easy to mistake low blood glucose for intoxication and delay treatment. Another concern is that while you're drinking, you may overeat or forget to check your blood glucose.

A mixed drink, beer, or glass of wine can fit in a diabetes food management plan, but only if you remember the following:

- Alcohol should be consumed with a regular meal or snack, not on an empty stomach.
- The quantity of alcohol should be limited to two drinks once or twice a week.
- Excessive alcohol consumption may impair your ability to recognize hypoglycemic reactions.
- Alcoholic beverages should be substituted for the appropriate food exchanges, or foods containing an equal amount of carbohydrates.
- Avoid sweet wines, liqueurs, sherry, and sweetened mixed drinks.

- When using such caloric mixers as fruit juice, the calories in the mixer must be counted.

- In cooking, alcohol evaporates and leaves only the flavor, so using it as an ingredient in the cooking process is fine.

- If you're having difficulty controlling your diabetes, skip the alcohol.

The Vegetarian Way

Not everyone eats from all areas of the Food Pyramid. Vegetarians eat a diet that's based on vegetables, beans and bean products, and such carbohydrates as potatoes, pasta, and breads. Ovo-lacto vegetarians also eat such animal products as milk, cheese, yogurt, and eggs. Vegans abstain from meat as well as eggs and dairy.

Vegetarians who happen to be diabetic can enjoy both a healthy life and their chosen eating style, but only if they follow a few basic ground rules.

A complete protein is a food that contains all essential amino acids. Animal proteins are classified as complete proteins; plant foods do not contain all the essential amino acids in proper quantities and are regarded as low-quality or incomplete proteins. By combining foods from any two of the following groups of vegetarian protein sources at the same meal, vegetarians can ensure they get essential amino acids:

- Soybeans.
- Dried beans, peas, and lentils.
- Grains, including oats, wheat, barley, rice, and corn.

- Nuts and seeds.
- Milk products.

These foods complement one another when eaten over the course of a day. Confirmed complementary proteins include grains and legumes, seeds and legumes, and grains with milk products. Typical dishes might include red beans and rice, nut loaf with corn, or cheese quiche with split pea soup.

Eating widely from the many alternative protein substitutes is one way to be sure you get the nutrition you need as well as the amino acids. That's where such protein substitutes as tofu, cheese, eggs, and nut butters come in.

Vegans need to include a source of vitamin B12 in their diets—for example, cereal or soy milk fortified with vitamin B12. In addition, if their exposure to sunshine is limited, a vitamin D supplement may also be needed.

When You're Sick

Whether it's a cold or a serious illness, a person with diabetes needs to take special measures when sick. Start by working with your health care team to develop a sick-day plan. That plan should serve as your guide for helping you get well and also include specific information about when to call the doctor.

In general, check your blood glucose levels according to the schedule outlined on your sick-day plan. If possible, eat normal meals. If you're too sick to eat, sip small amounts of juice every ten to fifteen minutes.

Diarrhea or vomiting requires further special attention, because you will be losing sodium and potassium, and fluids need to be replaced. Sodium can be replaced by adding salt to foods and by eating canned soup, broth, and salted crackers. Foods high in potassium include oranges, grapefruits, and vegetable juices; bananas; potatoes; and dried fruits. Many salt substitutes are also high in potassium.

6

The Vitamin Edge
· · · · · · · · · · · · · · · · · · · ·

The Program

What? Taking daily vitamins and mineral supplementation will add to the vitamins and minerals already found in a diet that is appropriate for a person with type 2 diabetes.

Why? A growing body of research shows that vitamin and mineral supplementation can improve the way your body responds to insulin. This research shows that vitamins with antioxidant properties lessen the impact of type 2 diabetes by "mopping up" free radical oxidants that occur as part of the disease process of diabetes and can damage nerves and blood vessels.

How? Make certain you are getting the recommended daily allowance (RDA) of the vitamins and minerals discussed in this chapter.

"Should I take more vitamins now that I have diabetes?"
"How much vitamin C is enough?"
"Are there enough vitamins in my food?"
These questions are asked of all medical doctors who treat people with diabetes. The answer the patient receives will be different, depending upon the bias of the doctor.

Many physicians recommend no vitamin supplementation at all. They feel that we get more vitamins and minerals in our daily diet than we need and shouldn't bother with extra pills.

Others take the "better safe than sorry" approach. Although they don't believe in vitamin and mineral supplementation, they don't disbelieve in it, either. To their way of thinking, a little extra supplementation won't hurt.

Others, like myself, heartily endorse the use of vitamin and mineral supplements. We have seen the positive effects of these supplements on patients with diabetes and know that they have virtually no side effects.

For many years Western medicine has been opposed to the taking of supplements. When I went to medical school the prevailing thought was that "health nuts" were the only ones who took supplements. We were encouraged not to recommend supplements to our patients. Some of the professors even felt that it amounted to quackery to do so.

Now things have changed. A growing body of medical research is showing that vitamins and minerals have a place in medicine, especially in the successful treatment of type 2 diabetes. This chapter focuses on that research and provides a clear path for you to follow in giving your body the essential nutrients it needs to battle diabetes.

Outside Influence

Vitamins and minerals, along with glucose, phytochemicals, and protein, as well as amino, fatty, linoleic, and linolenic acids, are the essential nutrients that your body doesn't make, but that you need to live a long, healthy life.

They are the foundation of good nutrition, because in their absence your body couldn't use the food you eat.

People with diabetes know that, along with exercise and following their medical team's recommendation regarding medication, getting the essential vitamins and minerals is one way to manage their disease successfully. Certain vitamins and minerals appear to pack a double punch for people with diabetes, because they may also have a role in lessening the risk of diabetic complications and may even help reduce the need for medication.

The use of vitamins, minerals, and other naturally occurring substances in food is the new frontier in the treatment of diabetes as well as in many other diseases. With in-depth research and continued study, scientists are unlocking the secrets these substances hold in disease prevention and management.

If you're one of the many people who think vitamins and minerals are the fuel that runs your body, think again. In fact, it's the calories in food that give you energy. Vitamins and minerals release that energy by allowing your body to digest, absorb, and metabolize nutrients. In essence, they are the key that, when turned, runs the engine of nutrition.

Thirteen vitamins essential to good health have been identified. These fall into two categories, water-soluble and fat-soluble. The water-soluble vitamins—C and the eight B vitamins—are found in the watery portions of food; they are absorbed directly into the bloodstream, circulating freely throughout the body. Fat-soluble vitamins—A, D, E, and K—can be absorbed only in the presence of fat. Fat-soluble vitamins enter the bloodstream via the intestinal wall. They are stored in fat storage sites in the body.

For the most part, the best way to maximize the nutritional potential of water-soluble vitamins is to eat as much of them as possible when they're fresh or frozen. Improper storage can lead to water-soluble vitamin loss. That's why it's important to store such foods, including citrus fruit, green vegetables, peppers, tomatoes, berries and potatoes, dairy products, liver and other organ meats, clams and oysters, eggs, fish, chicken, pork, whole-wheat products, brown rice, and oats carefully and in covered containers.

Avoid overcooking, as this can deplete the vitamin content. For instance, peas are an excellent source of thiamin, but if you overcook them, they can lose as much as 40 percent of their thiamin content. Milk is a good source of riboflavin, but that vitamin is sensitive to ultraviolet and fluorescent light. So milk stored in a clear container at the grocery store may have riboflavin depletion even before you take it home.

Minerals are the most basic element of nutrients. They can't be destroyed, unlike vitamins, which can be lost easily in cooking and storage. But that doesn't mean every mineral you take in is easily and immediately available to your body. Take spinach, for instance. It's packed with calcium, but most of the calcium is not available because it is bound to oxalic acid, and that blocks absorption.

At least sixteen minerals are identified as being essential to good health. Some are categorized as major minerals, others as trace minerals. The difference is in the amount the body needs, not in their importance to nutrition.

Medical research is only just beginning to uncover the delicate interrelationship between vitamins and minerals, and disease management and prevention. What we do know is that it's not enough simply to eat according to the Food Pyramid or even to take a daily vitamin supplement.

About Antioxidants

Everyone's talking about antioxidants. That's because preliminary epidemiological studies seem to show a relationship between these substances and disease prevention. The theory is that vitamins C and E, plus beta-carotene and other carotenoids, as well as the minerals selenium, copper, and manganese, may be instrumental in supporting good health through their actions in the body.

Antioxidants appear to protect cells from damaging oxygen-free radicals or oxidants. Oxygen-free radicals are released in the body as the result of the breakdown of food into fuel. These free radicals appear to damage cells in much the same way oxygen causes some metals to rust or oxidize.

This cell damage may be connected to a plethora of health problems, including heart disease, cancer, cataracts, and a weakened immune system, to name a few. In addition to the free radicals created as a natural part of the body's processes, most people also come into contact with free radicals through such external forces as tobacco smoke, pollution, and even rancid dietary fats. Remember that the next time you eat fast-food French fries that taste bitter, are exposed to secondhand smoke, or are tempted to leave your car idling while you run an errand.

Researchers at the Royal Brompton Hospital in London have linked abnormally high levels of blood glucose to the production of free radicals. They believe these free radicals may trigger a cascade of undesirable chemical reactions, leading to what they call "oxidative stress." The result? For people with diabetes, the potential for complications such as heart disease, blindness, kidney disease, and nerve damage.

Free radicals seem to wreak havoc on the body in a variety of ways. They appear to cripple the cell membrane, preventing it from taking in nutrients, oxygen, and water,and getting rid of waste products; they may even kill cells. They also may attack cells' genetic material, making it more likely to replicate and grow abnormally—essentially the disease process that makes cancer so deadly.

Fortunately the body has its own way of dealing with free radicals. To prevent their damaging effects, antioxidants step in. Some appear to control the free radicals; others seem to transform them into less damaging compounds; still others are believed to repair damaged cells.

Not all antioxidants are alike. In fact, they aren't interchangeable. Each has a unique job to do in nutrition and health. For instance, E may be most effective at protecting the arteries against heart disease and the prostate against cancers; carotenoids appear to guard the retina against degeneration.

Using an assay that measures isoprostane levels in urine, researchers at the University of Pennsylvania Medical Center have found a way to gauge oxidative damage caused by free radicals. This measuring system may become an integral tool in clearly understanding the action of antioxidants in protecting the body from free radical damage. Researchers continue to study the action of antioxidants in an effort to determine how they can be better harnessed to enhance disease fighting and prevention.

Phytochemical Facts

Phytochemicals are the new kids on the nutrition block. Classified as nonnutrient parts of food, phytochemicals are still being studied. What we do know is that they give plants their color and protect them from free radicals as well as viruses, extremes of heat and cold, and rough handling. Don't let the nonnutrient label fool you. While they have no calories and appear not to be crucial for normal function, researchers believe they are able to extend to people some of the same protection they give plants.

In animal studies, mice fed a diet of such food components as starch, protein, vitamins, and minerals were more likely to develop liver tumors than those fed whole foods. Phytochemicals are believed to act at three different points to prevent cancer—they seem to prevent cancer-causing substances from forming, boost the activity of blocking agent enzymes, and suppress precancerous activity.

Phytochemical Profiles

To date, researchers have identified only a handful of what are believed to be hundreds of phytochemicals. The existence and action of the remaining ones are still to be revealed. Some phytochemicals may hunt down free radicals, preventing LDL cholesterol from oxidizing and reducing the risk of heart disease and cancer. Here are just a few of the known phytochemicals, food sources, and believed roles in disease prevention.

- **Ellagic acid**. Common in grapes, strawberries, raspberries, and walnuts, this phytochemical appears to remove cancer-causing agents from the bloodstream.
- **Flavonoids**. A family of chemicals found in apples, red wine, and tea, flavonoids seem to play a role in

cancer and heart disease prevention. They may
reduce cancer risk by blocking hormones that
create cell changes and by suppressing changes in
malignant cells.

- **Indoles and isothiocyanates**. Cruciferous vegetables,
such as Brussels sprouts, cauliflower, and cabbage,
are especially good sources of antioxidant
phytochemicals.

- **Isoflavones.** Soybeans contain this phytochemical,
along with several other antioxidant substances,
including phytic acid, protease inhibitors, saponins,
phytoserols, and phenolic acid.

- **Lignans**. Commonly found in oil pressed from
flaxseed, lignans is a powerful antioxidant that also
contains omega-3 fatty acids that may protect
against heart disease and colon cancer.

- **Monoterpenes**. Commonly found in citrus fruits and
caraway seeds, this phytochemical can prevent
oxidation and keep potent carcinogens from taking
hold.

- **Organosulfur compounds**. Found in garlic, onions,
and other foods from the *Allium* genus, this
phytochemical has been found in studies to have a
possible impact on reducing the risk of colon and
stomach cancer.

- **Phenol**. Tea, especially green tea, is a good source of
phenol. It seems to activate enzymes that eliminate
oxidants.

Why a Pill Isn't Enough

Vitamins, minerals, and supplements are all the rage these days. From drugstore generics to pricey designer elixirs, you can buy a dizzying combination of substances, all of which claim to be indispensable in enhancing overall health, boosting energy, or resolving a particular deficiency.

The fact is, no pill or supplement can substitute for a balanced diet. A rich and varied diet containing fruits, vegetables, grains, dairy products and protein also includes fiber and phytochemicals essential for good health. A pill can't come close to supplying all those in the right combination or form, but when used to supplement the diet, appropriate formulas can be very helpful to the body.

Balance is another concern. Good nutrition is based on taking in appropriate amounts of vitamins and minerals to act on the calories you eat and burn through exercise. When you add large amounts of any one vitamin or mineral, you run the risk of disrupting this delicate balance.

There's also a risk of taking in, via a vitamin or supplement, a quantity that can damage your health. For instance, vitamin A is necessary for good vision, though too much can damage your liver. Taking large amounts of zinc because you heard it can augment your immunity could put you at risk for a copper deficiency.

The Food and Nutrition Board sets the recommended dietary allowances (RDAs) of vitamins and minerals. RDAs are guidelines for safe and adequate levels of nutrition, not optimal or even minimal requirements. That leaves room for individual need based on age, lifestyle, and health. Keep this in mind when you're studying food labels or considering the purchase of a vitamin or supplement.

The RDAs aren't dietary commandments. They don't dictate every substance each person needs for good health, because, in part, medical researchers are only now beginning to explore the intricate and individual relationships between vitamins, minerals, trace minerals, and other substances food supplies. Rather, RDAs are estimates based on the calculated dietary needs of healthy people whose food intake varies from day to day. If you have a chronic disease—high blood pressure, irritable bowel syndrome, or diabetes—you may need to append your diet, either with specific foods or with supplements, to make up for vitamins and minerals lost as a result of your disease or the medications you take.

Finally, RDAs don't take into account the changing nutritional needs that occur over a lifetime. For instance:

- Menstruating girls and women may need extra iron to compensate for blood loss during monthly flow.

- Women of childbearing years need extra folate before and during the first few weeks of pregnancy to reduce the risk of neural tube defects.

- Pregnant or breast-feeding women may need extra calcium, iron, and vitamin B6, plus folate to compensate for increased demands on their bodies.

- Adolescents and older men and women need extra calcium to build bone and prevent osteoporosis, *especially* if they have diabetes.

- Older adults, who are less active and less inclined to eat a balanced diet and whose bodies may not absorb nutrition efficiently, may need a multivitamin.

Whether you should be taking a multiple vitamin or specific supplements is a decision for you and your health care team to make based on your personal health, your lifestyle, and your age.

Diabetes: The Vitamin and Mineral Connection

Researchers increasingly are looking to vitamins and minerals as potential tools for treating people with diabetes. These substances may hold the key for long-term good health, complications management, and possibly even prevention.

Heart Disease

Cardiovascular disease is an ever-present concern for people with diabetes, who are at greater risk. According to the American Diabetes Association, adults with diabetes have heart disease death rates two to four times higher than adults without diabetes. At the same time, 60 to 65 percent of people with diabetes have high blood pressure; their risk of stroke is two to four times higher than that for people without diabetes.

University of Texas Southwestern Medical Center researchers described recent experiments in which people with diabetes and people without diabetes were given 1,200 international units of vitamin E daily. After eight weeks the process that leads to a buildup of fatty deposits in the arteries was slowed in both groups.

Therapy with vitamin C and other antioxidants shows promise in helping reduce the incidence of cardiovascular disease in some people with diabetes. The study, conducted at Brigham and Women's Hospital and Harvard Medical School, found short-term infusion of C improved blood vessel functions in ten patients with diabetes, but not in the ten who weren't diabetic.

The researchers studied the endothelium—the smooth layer of cells lining the inside of blood vessels, which helps them to dilate and contract properly. Previous research had indicated the endothelium could be damaged by oxygen-derived free radicals, while antioxidants such as vitamin C are believed to destroy these radicals.

Findings regarding vitamin E's antioxidant properties in preventing hardening of the arteries also are encouraging. In a study of middle-aged people who took vitamin E supplements, there was markedly less buildup of fatty plaque in the neck arteries than among test subjects who did not take supplements. Even among those who did not take supplements, the higher the person's dietary intake of vitamin E, the less arterial clogging.

The Nurses' Health Study, an ongoing investigation of many preventive health measures involving 70,000 female nurses, has shown a 50 percent drop in the risk of heart disease among participants who consumed high amounts of folic acid and B6. Folic acid and B6 are believed to interfere with the action of homocysteine, a chemical that worsens atherosclerosis. This study may have application in reducing risk, even though researchers endorsed good weight management and smoking cessation as the keys to the management of heart disease overall.

A study from the University of Maryland School of Medicine has found that consuming high doses of vitamins C and E before a high-fat meal may counter fat's ill effects. Researchers believe these vitamins somehow prevent triglycerides, a type of blood fat, from stopping blood vessels from releasing nitric oxide. Nitric oxide allows vessels to relax and widen, facilitating healthy blood flow to the heart.

Their study found that before a fatty meal, blood vessels could widen by 21 percent to accommodate the sudden rush of blood, but four hours after, could widen by only 8 percent. When study subjects consumed 1 gram of C and 800 international units of E before eating a high-fat meal, the amount by which their arteries could widen fell to only 17 percent four hours afterward.

Researchers believe the vitamins, which are antioxidants, squelch free radical action. Previous research has found that high cholesterol levels interact with oxygen in the body to produce an excess of oxygen-free radicals. These are known to interfere with nitric oxide and cause blood vessels to be less pliable. This impairment of blood vessels is a recognized risk factor for atherosclerosis.

Smoking Solutions

That smoking is linked to many types of cancer, high blood pressure, and cardiovascular disease is well documented. These associations are just some of the reasons people with diabetes are strongly discouraged not to smoke.

Researchers at the University of Freiburg in Germany and also at Boston University Medical Center have linked the taking of liquid vitamin C by smokers with impaired arteries to improved blood flow.

C is believed to clear from the body free radicals that smoking leaves behind. The free radicals damage endothelial cells, causing increased deposits of low-density lipoprotein (LDL), so-called bad cholesterol, and narrowing of the arteries. These two conditions can lead to heart disease and heart attack.

Calcium and Men

The positive effects of calcium in protecting women from osteoporosis, or "soft bones," is well known, but for men with diabetes, even a small shortage of calcium could increase their risk for the same condition. Osteoporosis is a leading cause of broken bones, debilitation, and death among the elderly (people sixty-five and older), 18.4 percent of whom have diabetes.

Researchers at Athens University Evangelismos Hospital tested thirty men and women with diabetes for bone loss in the spine and thigh. These measurements were then compared with those for people who did not have diabetes. They found that men with diabetes lost significantly more bone than men without diabetes over the course of the study. Diabetic women and healthy women lost bone at the same rate.

None of the women in the study were on estrogen replacement therapy, which helps to preserve bone strength. Diabetes experts hypothesize that because older women continue to produce small amounts of fatty tissue even after menopause, and many women with diabetes are overweight, they may be protected from osteoporosis.

The study is believed to refute the myth that people with diabetes have stronger bones because of their greater attention to good nutrition.

Vitamin and Mineral Know-How

Each vitamin and mineral plays a complex role in nutrition and overall good health. Use this guide to help you understand the jobs of each and their particular importance to people with diabetes.

Vitamins

Vitamin A—the eyesight vitamin. Especially important for people with diabetes, who are at increased risk for diabetic retinopathy, the leading cause of blindness among adults. Essential for vision and a strong immune system, vitamin A also helps build and maintain strong bones. Found in liver, fish liver oils, whole and fortified milk, and eggs, this vitamin can be synthesized from carotenoids, naturally occurring in orange fruits and some vegetables.

RDAs: Men—1,000 micrograms. Women—800 micrograms.

Possible negative effects of higher than recommended intake: Liver damage, as well as headache, vomiting, blurred vision, hair loss, flaking skin, bone and muscle pain, spontaneous abortion, and birth defects.

Beta-carotene—antioxidant. Converted as needed to make vitamin A. Good sources of this vitamin include spinach, collard greens, broccoli, carrots, peppers, sweet potatoes, apricots, and peaches. Through its antioxidant action, beta-carotene protects cells from free radical damage.

RDAs: Men—6,000 micrograms. Women—4,800 micrograms.

Thiamin—energy vitamin. Essential for people with diabetes, who may experience nerve damage as a complication for their disease. Thiamin acts as a coenzyme to get energy from carbohydrates, protein, and fat; it also converts excess carbohydrates to fat and is essential for initiation of nerve impulses. Good sources include yeast, lean pork, organ meat, legumes, seeds, nuts, and unrefined cereal.

RDAs: Men, nineteen to fifty—1.5 milligrams. Men, fifty-one and over—1.2 milligrams. Women, nineteen to fifty—1.1 milligrams Women, fifty-one and over–1.0 milligrams.

Riboflavin—hormone regulator. A must for the overall good health of people with diabetes. An active element in the release of energy from carbohydrates, fat, and protein, riboflavin is found in milk, yogurt, cottage cheese, meat, leafy green vegetables, and whole-grain or enriched breads and cereals. Essential for growth and development, riboflavin also regulates certain hormones and aids in the development of red blood cells.

RDAs: Men, nineteen to fifty—1.7 milligrams. Men, fifty-one and over—1.4 milligrams. Women, nineteen to fifty—1.3 milligrams. Women, fifty-one and over–1.2 milligrams.

Niacin—fat synthesizer. Since people with diabetes have a higher than average incidence of cardiovascular disease, getting enough niacin is important in minimizing the risk of heart disease. As a coenzyme that releases energy from carbohydrates, niacin is found in abundance in meats, especially liver, fish, legumes, nuts, whole-grain and enriched breads, and cereals.

Also found in coffee and tea, niacin is needed to break down fats and proteins, to synthesize fats and certain hormones, and to aid in red blood cell formation.

RDAs: Men, nineteen to fifty—19 milligrams. Men, fifty-one and over—15 milligrams. Women, nineteen to fifty—15 milligrams. Women, fifty-one and over–13 milligrams.

Possible negative effects of higher than recommended intake: Associated with gastrointestinal complaints, liver damage, aggravation of ulcers.

Biotin—carbon dioxide carrier. People with diabetes require biotin to help their bodies metabolize fat, since fat can contribute to coronary artery disease, one of the complications of diabetes. A coenzyme in energy metabolism that also carries carbon dioxide, biotin is found in liver, eggs yolks, soybeans, yeast, cereal legumes, and nuts. Used to synthesize fatty acids, biotin also assists in energy metabolism and the breakdown of certain amino acids.

RDAs: None established, but 30–100 micrograms is believed to be a safe and adequate daily intake for adults.

Pantothenic acid—diverse producer. A must-have for those with diabetes, who need to be exceptionally attentive to overall good health, especially eating a diet that's low in fat. While helping to metabolize fats, carbohydrates, and proteins, pantothenic acid, found in meats, whole-grain cereals, legumes, milk, vegetables, and fruits, also assists in the production of fats, cholesterol, bile, vitamin D, red blood cells, neurotransmitters and steroid hormones.

RDAs: None established, but 4–7 milligrams is believed to be a safe and adequate daily intake for adults.

Possible negative effects of higher than recommended intake: Associated with diarrhea, a condition for which many persons with diabetes already are at risk.

B6—multifaceted helpmate. B6's role in reducing the risk of heart disease makes it essential for people with diabetes. Fulfilling many essential nutritional roles, B6 helps to synthesize amino acids, nucleic acids, and red blood cells, and aids in the metabolism of proteins and urea. In combination with other B vitamins, B6, found in chicken, fish, kidney, liver, pork, eggs, brown rice, soybeans, oats, whole-wheat products, peanuts, and walnuts, may play a role in reducing heart disease risk.

RDAs: Men—2 milligrams. Women—1.6 milligrams.

Possible negative effects of higher than recommended intake: Nerve damage, a complication for which many people with diabetes are already at risk; also extreme sensitivity to light.

Folate—cell-growth vitamin. Another good source of vitamin support to aid people with diabetes in their fight against heart disease. By helping convert vitamin B12 to a coenzyme, folate assists in the synthesis of DNA in rapidly growing cells. In combination with folate and vitamins B6 and B12, folate may reduce the risk of heart disease. Folate is commonly found in yeast, organ meats, green and leafy vegetables, and some fruits. A lack of folate is linked to birth defects such as spina bifida, leading the U.S. Public Health Service to recommend that women of childbearing age get 400 micrograms of folate.

RDAs: Men—200 micrograms. Women—180 micrograms.

Possible negative effects of higher than recommended intake: Can mask symptoms of vitamin B12 deficiency and pernicious anemia.

Vitamin B12—another cell builder. Essential to the maintenance and replacement of cells and the nervous system, B12 supports the overall good health of diabetics, who are at greater risk for nerve damage. B12 plays a role in the metabolism of carbohydrates and fats, and the synthesis of proteins and certain amino acids. Found primarily in animal products such as organ meats, clams and oysters, milk products, other seafood, and eggs, B12, in combination with other B vitamins, may play a role in reducing heart disease.

RDA: 2 micrograms.

Possible negative effects of higher than recommended intake: According to the Harvard Medical School Health Group Publication on Vitamins and Minerals, no toxicity is reported for B12 at intakes up to 100 micrograms.

Vitamin C—the citrus vitamin. Even for those who can maintain good control of their diabetes, C is significant for its cell building and stress-management capacities. More than 80 percent of vitamin C in the U.S. diet comes from citrus fruits, green vegetables, peppers, tomatoes, berries, and potatoes. Its actions are diverse. It acts as an extracellular antioxidant to protect cells, regenerates oxidized vitamin E, and protects iron and promotes its absorption. Also commonly found in fortified breakfast cereals, it is essential to the formation of collagen and cell walls and helps the body deal with stress and illness.

RDAs: 60 milligrams. Up to 100 milligrams is recommended for smokers.

Possible negative effects of higher than recommended intake: May interfere with urine testing for diabetes and for blood in the stool; not advisable for people with a history of kidney stones.

Vitamin D—the sunshine vitamin. Some studies have shown that men who have diabetes are at increased risk for osteoporosis, and D may help protect them by helping to form and strengthen bones by making calcium and phosphorus more available. D also stimulates retention of these minerals by the body. Commonly manufactured by the body via exposure to the sun, vitamin D is found in fish liver oils, fatty fish, egg yolks, and fortified milk.

RDAs: Men and women, twenty-five and over—5 micrograms.

Possible negative effects of higher than recommended intake: Can cause damage to the cardiovascular system and kidneys, two complications that people with diabetes already face.

Vitamin E—cell protector. People with diabetes often experience dry skin; getting plenty of E can help alleviate that condition. Essential for normal cell structure and the formation of red blood cells, vitamin E is widespread in food. Best sources include vegetable oils, wheat germ, nuts, and green leafy vegetables. Also an antioxidant, vitamin E seems to protect the lungs and other tissues from damage by free radicals and pollutants.

RDAs: Men—10 milligrams. Women—8 milligrams.

Possible negative effects of higher than recommended intake: Impaired immune function and excess bleeding as well as gastrointestinal discomfort, a complication for which people with diabetes already are at risk; not recommended for people taking anticoagulants.

Vitamin K—clot creator. Diabetic kidney disease is the leading cause of people having to go on kidney dialysis. Since K is one of the vitamins that supports kidney function, it is fundamental for good health. Of the thirteen proteins essential for blood clotting, vitamin K contains at least six. Also playing a role in the synthesis of proteins found in plasma, bone, and the kidneys, vitamin K is widespread in food, including green leafy vegetables

RDAs: Men, twenty-five and over—80 micrograms. Women, twenty-five and over—65 micrograms.

Possible negative effects of higher than recommended intake: May cause a form of anemia, high levels of bilirubin in the blood, and jaundice in newborns.

Minerals

Calcium—bone builder. Getting plenty of calcium is vital for people with diabetes because of this mineral's important role in blood pressure regulation. It's also basic to bone formation and maintenance, and may play a role in reducing the precancerous changes in the lining of the colon. Found in milk, green leafy vegetables, tofu, sardines and salmon with bones, and calcium-fortified orange juice, calcium aids in blood clotting and nerve-impulse transmission.

RDAs: 800 milligrams.

Possible negative effects of higher than recommended intake: May inhibit the absorption of iron and zinc; very large amounts can lead to excess calcium in the blood and kidney damage, a concern for people with diabetes who are already at risk for kidney disease.

Chromium—metabolizer. Working with insulin to help cells absorb glucose and produce energy, chromium also supports carbohydrates, protein, and lipid metabolism. It is found in processed meats, whole-grain products, brewer's yeast, calf's liver, American cheese, and wheat germ.

RDAs: Up to 1,000 micrograms per day is recommended for people with diabetes, 150 micrograms per day for people without diabetes.

Possible negative effects of higher than recommended intake: Too much can result in stomach pain, cramps, and diarrhea.

Copper—energy resource. Copper is a part of an enzyme system that consumes oxygen or oxygen-free radicals that have been linked to cardiovascular disease, a complication of diabetes. Needed for energy and wound healing, copper is found in shellfish, nuts, seeds, legumes, organ meat, bran and germ portions of grains, as well as most grains, meats, mushrooms, tomatoes, bananas, grapes, and potatoes.

RDAs: 1.5–3.0 milligrams.

Possible negative effects of higher than recommended intake: Too much is associated with stomach pain, nausea, vomiting, diarrhea, coma, collapsed blood vessels, liver failure, and death.

Fluoride—tooth protector. Dental problems are common among people with diabetes, and fluoride can help with good dental hygiene. A beneficial mineral that protects against tooth decay, fluoride is available in tea, salmon and sardines with bones, and fluoridated water.

RDAs: 1.5–4 milligrams.

Possible negative effects of higher than recommended intake: Can impair bone health, a concern for men with diabetes who are at higher than average risk for osteoporosis. Also linked to kidney damage, another concern for people with diabetes who are already at risk for kidney disease; also impaired muscle and nerve function and linked to mottling of the teeth, nausea, diarrhea, chest pain, itching, and vomiting.

Iodine—regulator. At increased risk for nerve damage, people with diabetes need this mineral to maintain nerve and muscle function. It's also an integral part of two essential thyroid hormones and helps regulate growth and reproduction. Available in sea water and iodized salt, it also assists in the regulation synthesis of blood cells, body temperature, and the rate at which energy is released from nutrients.

RDAs: 150 micrograms.

Possible negative effects of higher than recommended intake: Enlargement of the thyroid gland.

Iron—oxygen transporter. Essential for overall good health, iron is basic for people with diabetes. By working with proteins to release energy in metabolism, iron helps carry oxygen in the bloodstream and muscles. Iron also is involved in making amino acids, hormones, and neurotransmitters and is found in meat, poultry, fish, fortified cereals, and some fruits and vegetables.

RDAs: Men, nineteen and over—10 milligrams. Women, nineteen to fifty—15 milligrams. Women, fifty-one and over—10 milligrams.

Possible negative effects of higher than recommended intake: Can cause nausea, vomiting, diarrhea, rapid heartbeat, weak pulse, dizziness, shock, confusion, and even death.

Magnesium—metabolizer. Another mineral that's crucial in the total health of people with diabetes, magnesium works in hundreds of chemical reactions in the body to metabolize food and transmit messages between cells. It's widespread in all unprocessed foods; good sources are nuts, legumes, whole grains, green vegetables, and bananas.

RDAs: Men—350 milligrams. Women—280 milligrams.

Possible negative effects of higher than recommended intake: Associated with nausea, vomiting, and low blood pressure. Very high concentrations can cause respiratory impairment, coma, and heart attack.

Phosphorus—another bone builder. Phosphorus has many functions that are fundamental to good health for people with diabetes, including bone and cell growth, maintaining the body's acid/base balance, releasing energy, and working with the transport of lipids in the blood and nutrients both in and out of cells. It's found in milk, meats, poultry, and fish, as well as legumes, fruits, alcoholic beverages, coffee, tea, and soft drinks.

RDAs: Men—1,200 milligrams. Women—800 milligrams.

Possible negative effects of higher than recommended intake: Irritation of the gastrointestinal tract, cramps, headache, and in extreme cases, liver and kidney damage.

Potassium—transmitter. For people with diabetes, potassium acts as a transmitter of nerve impulses and muscle contraction, and maintains normal blood pressure. The richest sources of potassium include unprocessed foods, especially fruits, many vegetables, legumes, and fresh meats.

RDAs: 2,000 milligrams.

Possible negative effects of higher than recommended intake: May cause muscle weakness, vomiting, and cardiac arrest.

Selenium—antioxidant helper. Selenium has many functions that are fundamental to good health for people with diabetes. Commonly found in seafood, kidney and liver meats, cereals, and grains, selenium is a component of an enzyme with antioxidant properties and may free vitamin E for other tasks.

RDAs: Men—70 micrograms. Women—55 micrograms.

Possible negative effects of higher than recommended intake: In very high doses can lead to nausea, diarrhea, hair loss, nail changes, irritability, fatigue, and nervous system disorders.

Sodium—volume regulator. Basic to nerve transmission, sodium plays a role in maintaining the good health of tissues at risk to damage from diabetes. Primarily a regulator of fluid volume, salt helps maintain acid/base balance in the body. Salt is integral to muscle contraction. Table salt is the best source.

RDAs: 500 milligrams.

Possible negative effects of higher than recommended intake: When taken over long periods, can lead to fluid retention and high blood pressure; the latter is a special concern for people with diabetes, who are already at risk for high blood pressure.

Zinc—metabolizer. Indispensable for people with diabetes because their disease may impair wound healing, a process zinc supports. A part of more than 100 enzymes, zinc plays a role in growth and development, immune function, blood clotting, wound healing, and sperm production. Available in meat, liver, eggs, and seafood, zinc also plays a role in the production of the active form of vitamin A in visual pigments.

RDAs: Men—15 milligrams. Women—12 milligrams.

Possible negative effects of higher than recommended intake: Linked to a lowering of copper levels. As a result, red blood cells shrink and immunity may be impaired. Gastrointestinal irrigation and vomiting also may occur.

More Than an Exorcist

A colleague once made the remark that he takes a multivitamin pill once a day because "it acts like an old-fashioned exorcist," preventing, even casting out, the effects of diabetes. Of course, research has shown vitamins and minerals to be more than superstition. In diabetics, adequate levels of vitamins and minerals have been proven to reduce blood sugar, lower blood pressure, improve vision, and get rid of free radical oxidants that damage cells and increase your chances of poor health.

Maybe my colleague was right. Taken in proper levels, vitamins and minerals can act as "exorcists" against the evils of diabetes.

7

De-Stressing for Diabetes Care
....

The Program

What? Use the stress reduction techniques recommended in this chapter before they are needed and when stress sneaks up on you.

How often? I recommend at least two concentrated sessions of stress reduction per day. That can mean performing your thirty minutes of exercise in the morning and a thirty-minute session of meditation in the evening. Stress reduction can be practiced at every opportunity during the day. If you feel yourself becoming stressed or angry, stop yourself, clear your mind by concentrating on your breathing, and count slowly to ten. This chapter offers a list of immediate interventions for stress reduction.

Why? Stress reduction intervention like meditation and even taking quiet "time-outs" has repeatedly been proven to lower blood pressure in test subjects. This is true even if the test subjects are heavy drinkers, are obese, consume excessive salt, or have diabetes. The lower your blood pressure (within reason), the less your chances of having complications of diabetes like heart disease or stroke. An immediate benefit of stress reduction is that it makes your life more pleasant immediately.

A "time-out" allows you to refocus on what is really important—namely, taking care of yourself.

I had an opportunity to see stress in action when a patient with diabetes, whom I will call Tim, came into an examining room at my clinic. He was tight with anger and didn't hesitate to tell me why.

"First I had one of those days at work," he said, scowling at me. "Then the traffic across the bridge was so heavy that I was late for our appointment. But I guess it didn't matter because when I got here I had to wait for nearly thirty minutes in the waiting room."

His speech had been explosive. When he finished he was panting from the increased heart rate his anger had caused. Beads of sweat covered his forehead, and his face was red from the high blood pressure that had resulted from the outburst. Before I could say anything, he looked at me with a blank stare and turned pale. Sitting down from dizziness, he was suddenly exhausted.

"I have to quit that," he said of his display of anger. "Diabetes and stress don't mix."

What Tim said was true. Although stress is a natural part of life, if you have diabetes, learning to avoid, anticipate, and manage stress is key in keeping your insulin levels under control and an essential part of living a normal, healthy life, despite your diabetes.

Some stress—taking a cranky four-year-old to day care when you're already late to work, while driving in rush-hour traffic during a thunderstorm—is obvious. But what about the anxious feelings you may get when you think about all your in-laws coming for dinner or that important presentation at work? Things don't have to be going badly for you to feel stressed. After all, the excitement of traveling to your child's college graduation or starting a new job can create the same physiologic reaction as negative stresses.

Many Forms of Stress

What people think is stressful is a matter of perception. Ask hospitalized patients what is currently stressful for them and they're likely to say, "Nothing, I'm not doing anything." In fact, just being in the hospital, having their regular schedules disrupted, and facing the specter of a new diagnosis or treatment are three very stressful factors. Though the second grade teacher may feel perfectly at ease amid twenty seven-year-olds, an options trader used to the heat of a trading session might break out in a cold sweat in a classroom with that same group of children.

Even socioeconomic status can produce stress. A recent study from the University of Michigan at Ann Arbor tracked 1,100 adults over age twenty-nine and measured the impact of a variety of indicators on personal health. They determined that the longer or more common episodes of hardship were in a person's life, the more severe the impact on health.

The skills you need for coping with different stressful situations are as varied as the stresses. You might be terrified at the idea of surfing, while the experienced surfer might be horrified at preparing a gourmet dinner for ten. Stress at work, in particular, can vary widely.

Richard Lazarus, a stress researcher at the University of California at Berkeley, makes a distinction between two kinds of coping. He describes emotion-focused coping, including talking out a problem or concern with a spouse or friends, to be most appropriate for such issues such as anxiety, pointless worrying, or a bad mood.

Problem-focused coping is more goal-oriented and includes intervention tactics that alter the path of threatening events or at least create potential strategies for alteration.

The trick is to develop your stress management skills, while distinguishing between the things you can control and those you can't, then taking appropriate action. Or at the very least, accept that it's out of your hands and move forward from there.

Stress and Diabetes

Stress causes real physiological and biochemical changes in the body, sometimes called the "fight or flight" response. In its simplest form, it works like this—you feel frightened and your body responds by releasing chemicals that make a quick escape possible. You can also call it the survival instinct, because it's the basic response that allows you to step quickly out of the way of a speeding car.

Even unexpected stresses that seem merely disruptive at the time—a flat tire or a surprise visit from a friend—can lead to jumps in glucose levels. Remember that the next time you test your glucose levels and find they're up, even though you've been dedicated to managing your diabetes well.

Most stresses aren't caused by matters of life or death. They're caused by matters of convenience or inconvenience, of personal preference, of deadlines, and of life's many demands and unmet expectations. When your body feels one of these, it activates the sympathetic nervous system and increases circulating levels of catecholamines, glucocorticoids, and growth hormones. These give your muscles and nerves the extra energy they need to respond by raising the level of blood glucose and ketones. Stress hormones also stimulate lipolysis, or fat breakdown. The release sends free fatty acids and glycerol into circulation to be oxidized into ketones.

In the person with diabetes, stress causes elevated blood glucose and ketones, because insulin doesn't work properly in them and allows glucose to rise. Research has found that people with diabetes differ from those without the disease in that they are particularly sensitive to these hormone responses. In their most severe reactions, that unplanned jump in glucose levels can even lead to ketoacidosis, which can cause diabetic coma.

Stress also may masquerade as hypoglycemia because many of the same responses occur in both situations. The result? Patients may misinterpret the symptoms of hypoglycemia—palpitations and shakiness—with psychological stress. The fear of experiencing hypoglycemia also can disrupt your daily life and add to your stress.

Illness is another form of stress that many people with diabetes underestimate. Whether it's a bad cold, recovering from surgery, or an ongoing battle with hay fever, the stress of illness can cause your body to release hormones that help you fight disease, but also make it difficult to control your blood glucose levels. That's why blood glucose monitoring is essential when you're sick. The best way to cope with the stress of illness is to talk with your health care team in advance to create a sick-day plan that helps you manage your diabetes during illness.

Sometimes a rise in glucose and difficulty in getting it back in control signals an undiagnosed illness or infection.

A Matter of Choice

You can't always control your hormones, but you can control the choices you make that *do* control your hormones. That's central to the idea that your type 2 diabetes is, for the most part, under your control and potentially curable.

Unfortunately, when some people feel stressed, they try to relax by drinking large amounts of alcohol, bingeing on junk food, cheating on sleep, or engaging in careless behavior, such as skipping meals. These behaviors may be benign for most people, but they can be deadly for those with diabetes. Each of these has the potential for increasing blood glucose levels, which are directly associated with a variety of dangerous complications, including depression and impotence, which can lead to further stress.

So what can you do? Take responsibility. Take time to assess and identify the stresses in your life. Then figure out which ones you can eliminate, and get to work. For the stresses you have to live with, create strategies that allow you to live with them and still manage your diabetes well.

That's where exercise can come in. When planned as a part of your regular diabetes management and with the support of your health care team, exercise is the single most effective way to reduce stress. Make exercise an integral part of your day. Do not wait until you can "find the time," but rather make the time, even if you do it in a passive way. For example, do your own yard work or even wash your car as ways of getting passive exercise. Exercise will fit most naturally in your life when it's a routine part of your day and involves activities you enjoy. (See Chapter 4, "Exercise That Fights Diabetes," to learn more about how exercise fits in with living well with diabetes.)

Mental Strategy for Stress

Some people just seem to be more stressed than others. That has to do in part with personality type and coping styles. Research has shown that "Type A" people, those who get angry or hostile when the pressure is on, tend to have higher glucose levels when they're under stress than "Type B" people, who are less inclined to let life's bumps and hassles affect them.

Though it's probably true that you can't change your personality, you can change the way you respond to stress. You must learn to solve problems instead of simply reacting and be proactive about stress management. Here are some techniques you can use the next time you feel stress mounting. Start by asking yourself:

- Is this life-threatening?
- What's the worst possible thing that could happen?
- Will this really matter next week? Next month? Next year?
- What can I realistically do now to alter how I feel?
- What's in it for me if I get angry, upset, anxious, whatever?
- What can I realistically do in the future to prevent this from becoming a problem again?

Many high-stress people set themselves up for a severe stress reaction, because they enjoy the "high" they get when their bodies engage in "fight or flight." They're impatient people who demand perfection from themselves and others. They overbook their schedules so they're always running late. Or worse yet, they don't keep a daybook of commitments, so they're always forgetting something important. They fail to schedule time to manage their diabetes, eat healthy meals, check their glucose levels, exercise, and relax. A Duke University study contends that people with diabetes who are under stress are five times more likely to die before the age of fifty than calmer, more trusting counterparts.

What you say and do are choices that affect not only how you feel, the quality of your life and your diabetes, but also other people around you. In *Love and Survival,* Dean Ornish writes about the choices we have in how we treat others.

I am finding that I have a choice in every moment to keep my heart open or closed, to live in love or in fear. More than any specific practice, I have found that maintaining this awareness of choice is the most important factor in keeping an open heart, for every action, every thought, every moment contains the potential for bringing us closer to either intimacy and healing or isolation and suffering. The direction is not inherent in the actions themselves but rather in the intentionality and motivation behind the actions.

The same hand that caresses also can kill. The same voice that soothes also can attack.

Make a change for the better by:

- Counting to ten before speaking up or taking action.
- Keeping a calendar of your commitments to others and yourself.
- Allowing an extra ten to fifteen minutes for every activity, especially those that depend on other people or require transportation time.
- Learning to say no to unreasonable or inconvenient requests or requests that in some way interfere with your diabetes management.

- Learning to say, "Yes, please," when help is offered.
- Following your diabetes management plan regarding diet, exercise, and monitoring.
- Keeping a diary of your blood sugar levels, food intake, exercise, and other activities that you can use to be proactive in stress management.
- Planning quiet time to rest and recoup.

Taking Time for Yourself

"I don't have time to relax."

It's a common complaint and sometimes a valid one. Your work, family, and community all make demands, but if you're not feeling your best, or if your blood glucose levels are above normal, you're actually cheating yourself and putting yourself at risk for life-threatening complications. Let the Diabetes Cure be your personal wake-up call to put your disease at the top of your priority list.

In *Anatomy of an Illness*, Norman Cousins wrote about his own encounter with disease. Through his experiences, Cousins discovered that hope, faith, love, and an abiding will to live, combined with a sense of purpose and a willingness to laugh (especially at himself), altered the quality and quantity of life.

His personal experiences were later supported by findings from Carnegie Mellon University, in which a study of 400 people found that psychological factors influenced the odds of fighting infection. Further, a Stanford University study determined that people with positive mental outlooks and strong social supports tend to take better care of themselves. They seek medical attention regularly, they eat nutritionally wholesome foods, and they bypass self-destructive behaviors like smoking, drug use, and alcohol abuse.

All of these behaviors are used to cope with daily stressors. You can replace any behavior with a different one if you have the will to do so. Realizing we are all creatures of habit, we need only make new habits.

The Art of Relaxation

Learning to relax is an art that must be cultivated and practiced. Relaxation can take many forms. For some people a quiet evening in front of the television is restorative. For others a round of golf, an afternoon in the garden, or praying quietly is refreshing.

Just conscious breathing can bring on relaxation and such benefits as lowered blood pressure, a slowed heart rate, and calm thinking. According to Robert Fried, a psychophysiolgist and author of *The Breath Connection*, the way most people breathe—rapidly and only expanding the upper part of the chest—leads to a chronic state of low-grade hyperventilation. The solution? Relearn how to breathe in a way that takes advantage of the diaphragm, the muscles separating your chest and abdomen. Consciously relaxing the abdominal muscles on the inward breath lets the diaphragm drop, opening up more space for the lungs. You'll know you have it right when your stomach bulges slightly as you inhale.

For people with diabetes, planning relaxation into the day is smart management and demands full and undivided attention. Here are some ideas.

Breathe with intention. Spending ten to twenty minutes to observe your breath is one of the best ways to restore body, mind, and spirit. Begin by loosening tight clothing and removing your glasses. Sit or lie in a comfortable position with your arms and legs uncrossed.

For a few moments, just follow your breathing with your mind's eye as it moves evenly in and evenly out. Gradually begin to lengthen the exhalation. So if you inhale to a count of four, exhale to a count of six, then eight, then ten, and so on. You may also wish to pause for a count of one or two at the bottom and top of the exhalation. If you feel breathless, return to normal breathing, then start again. If your mind wanders, try watching your breath while repeating to yourself: "I am breathing in. I am breathing out."

Change your thinking. Some people say, "As the mind goes, so goes the body." If you are inclined to see the dark side of life or are plagued by negative thoughts, those stresses are likely to show up in your body in the form of high blood glucose levels as well as headache, backache, stomachache, sleepless nights, and a host of other medical problems.

Changing lifelong thinking patterns demands diligence and practice. Pay attention to the negative thoughts you have and identify the activities and people who bring them out. Spend twenty minutes every day focusing on the positives in your life. Mentally revisit your favorite vacation spot. Focus your attention on a beautiful flower or photograph. Make a list of things that make you smile, then post that list on the fridge, the bathroom mirror, or your computer.

Keep a journal in which you intentionally list ten positive things each day. If negative thoughts emerge, acknowledge them, then refocus your attention on the positive. The notion that there is power in positive thinking may seem clichéd, but medical science shows that it can make a tremendous improvement in your health and happiness.

Relax progressively. This technique teaches you to recognize when parts of your body are tense and provides the awareness needed to relax them.

Begin by lying or sitting in a relaxed position. Focus on your right leg and tense all the muscles in it. Hold for five seconds and then release. Do the same with the left leg. Then move to the arms, abdomen, chest, neck, and head. Breathe slowly and deeply throughout and observe the contrast between tensed and relaxed muscles.

Laugh regularly and with gusto. Ever notice how much better you feel after a good laugh? Laughter facilitates the release of endorphins, brain chemicals that lift mood. Seek out opportunities that make you laugh, whether it's lunch with a friend, reading a funny book, or taking in a good movie. Cousins, during his illness, found Marx Brothers movies and *Candid Camera* reruns lifted his spirits and actually allowed him to cut back on pain medication.

Denial and Anger

Denial and anger can be elements or ingredients of stress. Together, they can make it difficult for you to stick with your diabetes management plan.

Denial is a common reaction to hearing the diabetes diagnosis, a change in your treatment plan, or the occurrence of a complication. Denial is a handy tool because it allows you to deal with bad news. It is easier to deny you have a medical problem, since it acts as a shield from the chronic nature of diabetes and its many complications. If you are pretending there is nothing wrong, those around you will do the same, and that doesn't help in the long run.

Anger is another element that can contribute to stress. The specter of complications or reactions, repeated trips to see your doctor, and the frustration of sticking with your care plan can leave you feeling angry and out of control.

Time for a Change

Start by talking with your doctor. Your physician may be able to determine if the way you feel is related to poor diabetes control or another factor. If your diabetes isn't well managed, your blood glucose may drop during the day, so your anxiety and fatigue may have a medical cause. These same low levels may cause you to eat too much. At night, low blood glucose can disturb your sleep. Working together, you and your doctor may be able to ease the stress, denial, and anger with a customized treatment regimen.

Support groups also can be a tremendous source of help. There you'll meet other people who have already faced the same issues. It's likely they will share ideas that helped them. Before adopting any idea that alters your treatment plan, be sure to talk with your health care team. Others can serve as the role models you need to get on track with your diabetes self-management.

Sometimes one-on-one counseling can make a difference. Whether you see a social worker, psychologist, or psychiatrist, these professionals can help you find new and healthier ways of living a full, rewarding life, despite diabetes.

Symptoms of Depression

Depression, whether it's the result of feeling a loss of control or directly the result of your diabetes, has specific symptoms. These include:

- Loss of energy.
- Inability to enjoy life.
- Increased appetite or weight loss.
- Trouble concentrating.
- Difficulty sleeping or changes in sleeping patterns.
- Memory lapse.
- Having trouble getting things done.
- Moodiness, irritability, or restlessness.
- Feeling empty or worthless.
- Suicidal thoughts.

Questionnaires are good tools to use in finding the source of problems like depression. The one that follows was developed by me and David MacDonald, D.O., a colleague who shares my interest in getting to the root of problems.

Solutions, Not Problems, with the 11-11 Scale

This scale focuses on eleven layers of interaction that exist between you and others. At any time you can take a quick "psychological temperature" or self-reading of where they are on the 11–11 Scale.

Although eleven points on all eleven scales is the ultimate target—121—points in all, most of us will never reach that level of satisfaction. Using this scale gives you an objective number to tell you how you are feeling at any point in time.

Take the test that follows. Answer spontaneously without thinking too much, since this should be a measure of your gut feeling.

An answer of 1 indicates that the way you feel about the question is poor, low, bad, couldn't be worse. An answer of 11 means that the way you feel about the question is great, excellent, couldn't be better. Try it for yourself and see how close to 121 you come.

Questions	Answers (1–11)
How do you feel about you, yourself?	_____
How do you feel about your soulmate?	_____
How do you feel about your family?	_____
How do you feel about your friends?	_____
How do you feel about your work?	_____
How do you feel about your environment?	_____
How do you feel about your spirituality?	_____
How do you feel about your nutrition?	_____
How do you feel about your physical activity?	_____
How do you feel about your level of control?	_____
How do you feel about your level of hope?	_____

··

Interpretation

11–30: You are probably experiencing conflict in many areas of your life, which can interfere with your overall health and wellness. If you score at this level for several days, you may consider seeking help from a professional trained in lifestyle management.

31–60: You probably have areas that are acceptable but many that are less than desirable. Look at specific low scores to see if there are any ways to bring the scores up. Perhaps your sense of control could increase if you increase the amount of exercise you do or improve your nutritional choices.

61–90: Your scores are more positive than negative, which means you are on the road to improved health and wellness. Keep trying to improve by identifying the low points and bringing them up.

91–121: If you fall into this range, keep up the good work. You probably have a good sense of what it takes to identify conflict and resolve it appropriately.

··

This scale not only gives you a total stress score, it also helps you isolate stressors in your life. If, for instance, you score yourself low on nutrition, then better eating would lower stress in your life. Or if you rate yourself low on your feelings about your family and also have a low sense of control, then family counseling might be the answer to reducing stress in your life.

The Language of Denial

Denial can be the greatest enemy to your long-term good health. Pay attention when you hear yourself say:

- "I feel fine. I know when my blood sugar is out of control."
- "I can't afford to see a doctor or dietitian."
- "It doesn't matter if I skip testing my blood glucose today."
- "That looks good, a little more won't hurt me."
- "It's too much trouble to test my blood sugar at work."
- "That sore on my foot will heal."
- "I can't be bothered cooking separate meals for my family and me."
- "I smoke or I drink alcohol. It's who I am and I'm not giving it up."

Finding and pursuing fulfilling activities is important for everyone, but especially for the person with diabetes. Here are some ideas about how to turn your attitude and life onto a more positive path:

- Make new friends and nurture old friendships. People who interact in a positive way with others tend to live longer, happier lives.
- Foster family ties and traditions. Seek ways to build continuity and support in your life through family and family traditions.
- Get involved. Join a community group, volunteer, help out, and reach out. The more you think of others, the less likely you are to feel sorry for yourself.
- Get busy. Pursue a hobby that you enjoy and that allows you to interact with others. Sign up for a class. Learn or teach someone else a new skill.

- Get fit. Talk with your doctor about appropriate fitness activities.

At Work

Your work is a part of who you are, and so is your diabetes. One Swedish study in the *Journal of Occupational Medicine* found that the amount of support from supervisors and coworkers, and the ability to control the pace, volume, and type of work all play into the amount of stress you feel at work. The same study found a connection between repetitive and monotonous work and workers' difficulty in relaxing, even after the workday ended.

Exactly how much your diabetes affects your work life is very individual. Some factors include:

- Your hours. Do you work shift work or 9 A.M. to 5 P.M.?
- Your work style. Does your work easily accommodate snacks, breaks, and checking your glucose levels?
- Your work environment. Are the people you work with a supportive team, or is it each person for himself or herself?
- Your profession. Does your work allow you some control over the amount of work you have?
- Your benefits. Does your job have such benefits as insurance that make proper managing of your diabetes possible?
- Job satisfaction. Do you love your job or profession, or is it just a paycheck? Is it rewarding and satisfying? Do the pay and benefits meet your needs?

Depending upon how well controlled your diabetes is, the disease may or may not be an issue at work. Talk with your diabetes management team about your employment. Keep careful records of your blood glucose levels and work activities. If appropriate, talk with your boss about changes at work you may need to make to maintain your job performance while managing your diabetes.

Constructive Ways to Cope with Stress

- Exercise.
- Relaxation.
- Hobbies.
- Visualization.
- Therapy.
- Spirituality or faith.
- Support groups.

Destructive Ways to Cope with Stress

- Skipping meals or overeating.
- Using too much alcohol or prescription medication.
- Using illicit drugs.
- Skipping appointments with your health care team.
- Holding your feelings in.
- Isolating yourself.
- Abusing family and friends.
- Not exercising.

On the Road

Travel, whether for business or pleasure, can present specific challenges for people with diabetes. The excitement of preparation and planning, visiting new places, meeting new people, and eating out can cause your blood glucose to rise. Likewise, changing time zones and schedules can make diabetes management difficult. Talk with your doctor about any special considerations you may have and use these tips to help you feel the best while on the road.

- Keep your diabetes supplies with you at all times. Never check them with baggage. Pack twice as much as you normally need in case of delays or an emergency.

- Carry snacks and glucose tablets (and in some countries, purified water) with you at all times. This is especially important if your travel schedule is a rigorous one.

- Talk with your doctor about adjusting your food plan to accommodate time zone shifts and regional differences in food.

- Wear your diabetes identification at all times.

- Take at least two pairs of shoes that are comfortable and well broken in. Change your shoes and socks at least once a day and take extra care in checking your feet for abrasions, blisters, and chafing.

- If traveling in countries where English isn't commonly spoken, learning how to say a few basic phrases can be a life saver. For example: "I am a diabetic." "Please get me a doctor." "May I please have sugar or a glass of orange juice?"

The International Association for Medical Assistance to Travelers (IAMAT) has set up centers in twenty-five countries staffed with English- or French-speaking physicians who are on twenty-four-hour call. IAMAT also publishes a directory of medical centers and associated physicians who have agreed to a set payment schedule for IAMAT cardholders. The organization also can provide information about food, climate, and sanitary conditions in countries you plan to visit. For more information, call 716–754–4883.

8

An Ounce of Prevention

The Program

What? Live with the confidence of a person who knows he or she will not get type 2 Diabetes.

How? By following a five-step prevention program:

- Step 1: Know your risk of type 2 diabetes.
- Step 2: Watch your weight.
- Step 3: Eat from a healthy list of body-friendly foods.
- Step 4: Exercise on a daily basis with activity you enjoy.
- Step 5: Take HCA as a prevention against type 2 diabetes.

When? Think about these steps to prevention every day to make changes easier.

Why? Because type 2 diabetes can be prevented, controlled, and *cured* using these five simple steps.

Prevention is the best medicine, especially when it comes to type 2 diabetes. Researchers and medical professionals have identified the following as essential to preventing or lowering your risk of developing diabetes.

BOX 8.1

A CHART REVIEW OF 353 PATIENTS IN A LARGE CALIFORNIA HMO REVEALED THERE IS A SERIOUS LACK OF PREVENTIVE CARE IN DIABETES PATIENTS . . .

- 56% of patients had no HbA1c.
- 39% who had HbA1c were over 10% (i.e., blood glucose greater than 250).
- 65% had no fasting blood sugar (FBS).
- 76% had no lipid measurement.
- 52% had no urinary protein measurement.
- 78% had no ophthalmology referral.
- 94% had no foot exam.
- 45% had an emergency department visit for diabetes.

It Is Important to Keep Checking the Following Regularly:

- Hemoglobin A1-c (HbA1c) every 3 months
- Fructosamine (glycoprotein) testing every 3 to 4 weeks.
- Assure that blood glucose is less than 250.
- Fasting blood sugars.
- Measurement of serum lipids.
- Ophthalmological referral for retina examination yearly.
- Careful foot exam—podiatrist recommended yearly.
- Prevention and education to avoid ER visits unless necessary.

Source: A. L. Peters, "Quality of Outpatient Care to Diabetic Patients: A Health Maintenence Organization Experience," *Diabetes Care* 19(6), 1996; 601–606.

Know your risks for developing diabetes. Have your blood glucose level checked regularly. After age forty-five, have it checked every three years, more often if the resulting reading is high or if you have a family history of diabetes.

Those at higher risk—Native Americans, African Americans, and those of Hispanic and Asian descent—should be tested earlier and more often.

Keep your weight in a range normal for your height and age.

Eat a well-balanced diet that is low in calories, fat, and refined carbohydrates.

With your physician's approval, develop an exercise program including twenty to thirty minutes of aerobic activity daily, plus stretching and strengthening activities.

Take HCA preventively as a means of improving your insulin receptivity. This will help you lose weight, and it will help you feel more energetic, which will make exercise easier and more desirable to do.

Experts estimate that almost all type 2 diabetes could be avoided, controlled, or *cured* by following these guidelines. Although more and more people are becoming sedentary and overweight, nationwide surveys have shown fewer risk factors for diseases like type 2 diabetes in populations educated about safe lifestyles. By reading this book, you know how to make yourself healthier and are more likely to do it. Congratulations! By following these steps, you will lead a happier and healthier life. You will also help friends and family make changes that will improve their lives, too.

Let's take a look at each of these steps to wellness.

Step 1: Know Your Risk of Type 2 Diabetes

About one in seventeen Americans, or 6 percent of the population, has diabetes. Every year 655,000 new cases are diagnosed, with 90 to 95 percent of those among people over twenty with type 2 diabetes. Half of these are unaware they have diabetes. That's because it's possible to have mild symptoms for years before finally seeking medical help. Symptoms of type 2 diabetes include:

- Unusual thirst.
- Frequent desire to urinate.
- Blurred vision.
- Frequent, prolonged fatigue with no apparent cause.
- Leg pain.
- Unexplained weight loss.

Most people with type 2 diabetes are insulin-resistant. That means, although their pancreas is producing insulin, either their cells are unable to obtain it or insufficient insulin is being produced. No matter what the cause, without insulin's effect to meet your body's needs, glucose levels rise and diabetes and its many complications can result.

The Gene Connection

The link between a family history of diabetes and your risk of developing it is clear, but not necessarily inevitable. The link is certainly stronger for type 2 than type 1. Researchers have yet to identify and isolate a single type 2 diabetes gene. What they do know is that if you have type 2 diabetes and are an identical twin, there is a 60 to 75 percent chance your twin also will develop the disease.

The high incidence of diabetes among certain minority groups also supports the genetic connection. African Americans, Asian Americans, Pacific Islanders, some Hispanic Americans, and Native Americans all get diabetes more often than Caucasians. Native Americans have the highest rate of diabetes in the world, and Mexican Americans, who share genes with Native Americans, have higher rates than Cuban Americans, among whom less intercultural breeding has occurred.

Some researchers believe the same genes that cause obesity may play a role in diabetes. Scientists compared the Arizona Pima Indians with the Mexican Pima Indians, two tribes related by genetics but separated by culture and national borders. The Arizona Pimas live thirty miles south of Phoenix on a reservation with electricity, running water, televisions, and cars. Many are unemployed, and most of those who do work have sedentary jobs. Their diet, like that of many Americans, is heavy on fatty, processed food.

The Mexican Pimas, on the other hand, live in the Sierra Madre mountains of Mexico. They have no electricity or running water. They have no modern conveniences, and all jobs require heavy physical labor. Their traditional diet is very low in fat and incorporates lots of beans and handmade tortillas.

When scientists compared the two groups' diabetes risks, the difference was startling. Scientists found while Mexican Pimas and their non-Pima neighbors had similar rates of diabetes—6.4 percent versus 3.4 percent—the rate for Arizona Pimas was 38.2 percent. Scientists peg the increased diabetes risk in Arizona Pimas to obesity.

The University of Washington developed this analysis to help you calculate your risk of developing diabetes. Test yourself on with following questions and scores:

••

I had a baby weighing more than nine pounds at birth or had diabetes during my pregnancy.
If yes, score 6. If no, score 0.

I have a parent, sister, or brother with diabetes.
If yes, score 3. If no, score 0.

I am Hispanic, African American, Native American, Asian American, or Pacific Islander.
If yes, score 3. If no, score 0.

I am overweight.
If yes, score 3. If no, score 0.

I have been told I have a high blood sugar level.
If yes, score 6. If no, score 0.

I am between 45 and 64.
If yes, score 1. If no, score 0.

I am under 65 and I get little or no exercise during the usual day.
If yes, score 3. If no, score 0.

I am 65 or older.
If yes, score 3. If no, score 0.
••

Total your score and check your risk.

If you scored 1 to 5 points you probably are currently at a low risk of developing diabetes. If you scored 6 or more, you are at high risk of having or getting diabetes.

Other Causes for Concern

There are other causes of type 2 diabetes not covered in this test. Recent research has linked chemical exposure and the use of certain medications to type 2 diabetes and other forms of diabetes as well. Exactly why this happens isn't known, but medical science is working hard on that question as you read this book.

Several studies have pointed to a connection between dioxin, a deadly chemical once used worldwide in pesticides and the defoliant Agent Orange, and diabetes. One study compared the occurrence of diabetes among Vietnam veterans who were exposed to Agent Orange during duty in Vietnam with those who had not been exposed.

The exposed veterans were 50 percent more likely to develop diabetes. Another study points to a possible link between dioxin and the startling jump in type 2 diabetes among children around the world. Researchers speculate a connection between obesity, diabetes, and the body's storage of chemicals such as dioxin in fat cells.

People who take protease inhibitors, a powerful new drug to treat people with AIDS, appear to have an increased risk of diabetes. The actual risk of diabetes from protease inhibitors is not known because many of the estimated 150,000 HIV-positive Americans on the drug may have undetected hyperglycemia. The Food and Drug Administration speculates the risk is between 1 in 100 and 1 in 1,000.

Contraceptives and Pregnancy

The jury is still out on whether the use of oral contraceptives contributes to the development of diabetes. One study at the University of Southern California Medical School found those who have had gestational diabetes or had a family history of diabetes and take certain birth control pills after delivery may triple their risk of developing diabetes later in life.

The women at greatest risk for developing type 2 diabetes years later used the suspect contraceptives for six months to a year after deliveries complicated by gestational diabetes, according to a study that focused on almost 1,000 obese Hispanic women who recovered from gestational diabetes four to six weeks after delivery. Over the next seven years, 56 percent of the women used some form of hormonal contraception. The contraceptives identified as producing the greatest risk of type 2 diabetes were progestin-only pills, progestin implants (Norplant), and estrogen-progestin combinations with the strongest progestins.

A different study from Harvard Medical School placed the blame squarely on obesity. Women who have diabetes or who are at risk for developing it—either through a previous gestational diabetic episode or a history of diabetes in their families—should talk with their doctors about taking combination contraceptives with the lowest dose and potency of progestin. Of the contraceptives studied, the combination pill containing norethindrone (0.40 milligrams) appeared to be the safest and did not appear to increase risk.

Step 2: Watch Your Weight

The number of Americans with type 2 diabetes has been increasing dramatically. It has jumped almost 50 percent since 1983 and tripled since 1958. In 1958 less than 1 percent of the U.S. population had diabetes. Today that percentage is 3 to 4 percent, according to the National Institute of Diabetes and Digestive and Kidney Diseases.

The International Diabetes Institute predicts the number of people with diabetes worldwide is expected to double by 2010. Diabetes has been called epidemic in many regions of the world, especially the West. Currently 123 million people worldwide have diabetes. By 2010 the figure is expected to grow to 220 million. Experts point to increasing weight and sedentary lifestyles as the catalysts.

About nine of ten people with type 2 diabetes are overweight. According to the World Health Organization, by the year 2025 more than 300 million adults worldwide are expected to have diabetes. Insulin resistance seems to be the cause. Insulin resistance—the body's failure to respond to insulin—develops as weight increases. Experts believe that at least 80 percent of type 2 diabetes could be eliminated by getting rid of obesity.

Losing as little as ten pounds and keeping it off can cut your risk of developing diabetes. Modest weight loss works even for those who would otherwise be at high risk of developing the disease, a study from the University of Pittsburgh has shown. The study focused on 157 overweight men and women between the ages of thirty-nine and fifty-five, all of whom had at least one parent with type 2 diabetes, though none of them showed signs of having diabetes.

After six months scientists found every participant who made lifestyle changes and lost weight had a reduction in average blood glucose levels. In fact, researchers calculated that a ten-pound weight loss maintained for two years could reduce risk of developing diabetes by 31 percent. Where you carry weight also seems to be a factor in developing diabetes. Extra weight above the hips is riskier than fat in the hips and thighs.

As everyone knows, losing weight is moderately easy. Keeping it off is tough. Yo-yo dieting—losing and regaining weight—appears to be another factor increasing the risk of developing type 2 diabetes. In a study published in *Obesity Research*, rats on a yo-yo diet that alternated adequate caloric intake with severe caloric restrictions developed insulin resistance as they aged, a precursor of type 2 diabetes. Instead of yo-yo dieting, the answer is to make slow, permanent weight loss your goal via a low-fat diet and regular exercise.

Not just adults are at risk. Children as young as eight are developing type 2 diabetes, and at an increasing rate. Researchers at the Arkansas Children's Hospital tracked fifty children with type 2 diabetes and compared them with fifty kids with type 1 diabetes.

Type 2 children, researchers found, were nearly all obese; more than 30 percent already had high blood pressure. Of the children with type 2 diabetes, 74 percent were black and 24 percent white. In contrast, 18 percent of the type 1 children were black and 82 percent white, a statistical makeup not unlike the demographics of Arkansas's population.

The finding startled researchers because type 2 diabetes usually develops in people over thirty, and previously was considered rare in children. Type 2 diabetes is associated typically with obesity, and the latest figures show obesity in children and teens has increased dramatically in recent years.

This is not the first study to uncover rising rates of type 2 diabetes in children. Two studies in San Diego and one in Cincinnati came to similar conclusions about children in those areas, suggesting this is a nationwide phenomenon; some experts speculate it may even be worldwide. At a recent meeting of the International Diabetes Federation Congress in Helsinki, Finland, experts agreed that the world faces a global explosion in diabetes unless people who are obese can lose weight.

Body Weight for Adults

Keeping your weight in a range normal for your height and age is the single most important thing you can do to reduce your risk of diabetes. The following are recommendations from the U.S. Department of Agriculture.

Height in Inches No Shoes	Weight in Pounds Without Clothing	
	Age 19–34	Age 35 and Over
5'0"	97–128	108–138
5'1"	101–132	111–143
5'2"	104–137	115–148
5'3"	107–141	119–152
5'4"	111–146	122–157
5'5"	114–150	126–162
5'6"	118–155	130–167
5'7"	121–160	134–172
5'8"	125–164	138–178
5'9"	129–169	142–183
5'10"	132–174	146–188
5'11"	136–179	151–194
6'0"	140–184	155–199
6'1"	144–189	159–205
6'2"	148–195	164–210

6'3"	152–200	168–216
6'4"	156–205	173–222
6'5"	160–211	177–229
6'6"	164–216	182–234

SOURCE: USDA, Department of Health and Human Services, *Dietary Guidelines for Americans*, 1990.

Step 3: Eat from a Healthy List of Body-Friendly Foods

Mounting evidence suggests diets low in fiber and high in the "wrong" carbohydrates—refined items such as white bread and granulated sugar—more than double the risk of developing diabetes.

According to a large prospective study, different foods trigger different amounts of insulin secretion, even if the foods contain the same amounts of carbohydrate. The difference (glycemic index) lies in how easily the starch is digested. White bread and mashed potatoes are very digestible and lead to substantial insulin secretion; dark bread, yogurt, and fruits are less digestible and trigger less insulin. Eating too many of the wrong carbohydrates too often can lead to elevated insulin levels, a risk factor for diabetes. To lower your risk of developing diabetes, the less refined the food you eat, the better, researchers say.

Everyone knows fiber is good for you. Lack of dietary fiber has long been considered a risk for several chronic diseases, including diabetes. Researchers fortified this link by following more than 65,000 women over six years. Taking into account obesity, sedentary lifestyles, genetics, and other risks, the results show fiber intake, especially cereal fiber, reduces the incidence of diabetes. Fruits, vegetables, and grains, especially unrefined cereals, are excellent sources of "good" fiber—unrefined carbohydrate, fiber, and some magnesium.

A study from the Netherlands found that men who ate healthy meals and exercised were less likely to develop insulin resistance. Researchers, working with 389 elderly men who did not have diabetes, found insulin levels were highest among those who got the least exercise and whose diets included the largest proportion of saturated fats and alcohol. High insulin levels are a sign of insulin resistance. Insulin levels decreased as the amount of high-fiber carbohydrates increased. Insulin levels also declined in men who consumed fats as polyunsaturated oils.

Another study, this one from Stanford University, found that subjects who took three to five times the recommended daily average of vitamin A were 40 percent better able to move glucose from their blood to their cells.

Vitamin A is a fat-soluble vitamin commonly found in liver, fish liver oils, whole and fortified milk, and eggs, as well as in orange fruits and vegetables and green leafy vegetables. It's essential for vision, a healthy immune system, and bone building. Because of the health risks associated with overdosing on vitamin A supplements, it's a smarter strategy to maximize your intake of vitamin A-rich foods.

Step 4: Exercise on a Daily Basis with Activity You Enjoy

Exercise—almost any kind of exercise—can reduce your risk of developing diabetes. Whether you're a dedicated swimmer or walker, a serious gardener or a frequent stairs-instead-of-the-elevator person—getting active and staying active pays off.

Don't be confused. Being physically active isn't the same thing as fitness. According to researchers at Johns Hopkins University, it isn't necessary to devote your life to physical fitness to gain health benefits. Their research has shown a reduced disease risk comes with just modest amounts and intensity of exercise—as little as thirty minutes of activity per day.

Here's an example of how that thirty minutes can pay off. The Honolulu Heart Program studied 6,815 men, looking for a link between exercise and diabetes. The men, who were diabetes-free when the study began, provided detailed information about their lifestyles, including their exercise programs and day-to-day activities, such as walking or gardening.

Six years later researchers found diabetes developed most frequently in those who were the least active. Compared with the active men, the inactive men's risk of developing the disease was 51 percent greater.

For older adults, who make up a substantial portion of persons with diabetes, regular, physician-approved activity may be even more beneficial than dietary changes in reducing the risk of developing diabetes, according to the University of Washington. An estimated 18.4 percent of people sixty-five and older have diabetes.

The good news about increasing your activity level is that many people see quick improvement of insulin resistance. A University of Michigan study found that one hour a day of walking or stationary bicycling reduced the insulin resistance of seven of eleven African-American women.

Take note—"activity" is different from the single-minded pursuit of strong biceps, four-minute miles, or rock climbing. To improve your health, your goal should be to incorporate thirty minutes of accumulated activity every day. The payoff is broader than just lowering your risk of developing diabetes. It also includes the potential to lower your blood pressure; reduce your risk of cardiovascular disease and osteoporosis; and help you sleep better, think more clearly, and feel less stressed.

With regular activity comes an increase in muscle mass. The greater the percent of muscle, the more effectively you burn calories in food and the more sensitive your body is to insulin.

Step 5: Take HCA As a Prevention Against Type 2 Diabetes

In theory, type 2 diabetes is easy to prevent because it is largely a disease of lifestyle. That means simply that this disease can be caused by the habits you have developed in your life, especially ones that make you eat too much and exercise too little. Following the Diabetes Cure program *even if you don't have diabetes* means that you are changing these habits and preventing diabetes and many other diseases of lifestyle. By following the simple plan outlined in this chapter, for example, you can prevent such afflictions as heart disease, strokes, arthritis, gout, and possibly even some forms of cancer. The National Institutes of Health says that six out of ten diseases are caused by lifestyle and would never have happened if diet, exercise, and other lifestyle guidelines had been followed.

Taking HCA in the amounts recommended in this book and following the exercise and diet guidelines will help you lose weight, which is the number one cause of type 2 diabetes. If you weigh too much for your height, as indicated by the height/weight chart in this chapter, consider following this program as a preventative measure against diabetes and as a means of improving overall health.

"Unteaching" Habits

If so many diseases are so easy to cure, why are afflictions like type 2 diabetes on the rise? The answer lies in habit control. Our habits have been with us our entire lives and some even longer, when you consider that they were handed down to us by our parents. So the children of vegetarians usually grow up to become vegetarians, just as meat-eating families spawn meat-eating children.

It is difficult to change the habits with which we were raised because they are what we know and are part of our identity. Many people have guilt about their habits, especially those who are overweight. They, more than anyone, would like to change their habits and lose weight, but it requires a constant vigilance that they sometimes cannot maintain.

Frankly, it is difficult enough to make lifestyle changes without feeling guilt about failing. I have had patients cry in my treatment rooms because they have failed to maintain an exercise program or to avoid their favorite fattening foods. I'll tell you what I say to them. "Our habits have been taught to us by many people throughout the years. We learned to eat too much ice cream from someone just as we learned to sit in front of the television from someone. Lifestyle change and habit control is a long, slow process that takes time. Ask your family and friends for help and ask them to be understanding." As far as I am concerned, slow and realistic change is the only way to make lifelong lifestyle changes.

9

Diabetes Disease Review

Diabetes affects more than your blood glucose levels. It's a chronic condition that, when left unchecked or poorly managed, can devastate virtually every organ and system of the body.

It can be difficult to understand and accept that what you eat today, the amount of exercise you get this week, and how you manage your diabetes with a program like the one outlined in this book can make a difference in your health. But it's true. Every day of diligent blood glucose control, of a balanced diet plus exercise, is an investment in reducing the risk of complications and improving your potential for long-term quality of life.

For many years medical professionals were able to see the benefits of diligent diabetes control in their patients. It wasn't until the close of the Diabetes Control and Complications Trial in 1993, however, that research and study supported and confirmed this intuition.

Study participants who maintained rigorous control of their glucose cut their complication risk in half. They had 76 percent less eye disease, 60 percent less nerve damage, and 35–56 percent less kidney damage. Researchers believe people with type 2 diabetes can reap similar benefits from tight blood glucose control coupled with lifestyle changes such as weight loss and exercise. The benefits of tight control were so obvious that the study was ended early and the findings announced so that others could benefit from them, too.

Changing for the Better

Even if you already are experiencing some diabetes complications, take heart and take action. Strict blood glucose control and smart lifestyle choices can minimize complications and may prevent the development of additional ones. Those who feel tight control just doesn't work for them can still reduce the risk of developing life-threatening complications by keeping their weight under control, exercising, and managing their disease.

The fact is, nearly every complication of diabetes comes from having too much glucose in your blood. A good metaphor is what happens when you put lots of sugar in a glass of tea or cup of coffee. The beverage becomes sticky and thick. That same dynamic is at work in most diabetes complications.

The thickness causes arteries and veins to narrow and blood flow to be reduced. It also can damage nerve cells and interrupts or stops electrical messages, such as sensations of pain or heat that your cells send to all parts of the body. Without sufficient or smooth system-wide blood flow or in the absence of efficient nerve conductivity and performance, a wide range of complications from atherosclerosis and heart attack to blindness, impotence, and nerve damage can occur.

Complications Overview

The complications of diabetes are diverse and widespread. Some are common and well known and many are related. Others occur on a limited basis, often in the presence of preexisting complications. Here's an overview of the most frequently experienced diabetes complications, how you can prevent them, and some of the common methods of treatment.

Hypoglycemia

The possibility of hypoglycemia is a part of having diabetes, especially if you use insulin or other diabetes medications. It occurs most often before meals, when insulin is peaking, or during or after vigorous exercise. You can even experience hypoglycemia when you're asleep. It can be especially problematic for pregnant women.

When blood glucose levels drop too low, you can feel dizzy and shaky. If untreated, you can lapse into unconsciousness, have seizures, and go into a coma. This is a true medical emergency that can be life-threatening if left untreated. Symptoms include:

- Weakness or fatigue.
- Rapid heartbeat.
- Shaking and sweating.
- Dizziness and impaired vision.
- Hunger.
- Headache.
- Loss of coordination.

- Nausea.
- Nightmares.
- Irritability, anger, and confusion.

A severe occurrence can leave you so disoriented or belligerent that you can't help yourself or even ask for help from others.

These symptoms may be misinterpreted as drunkenness, drug abuse, or a psychiatric disorder. That's why it's important to work to avoid hypoglycemia as well as to wear diabetes identification, so that your condition can be spotted and treated, even if you can't speak for yourself.

People who take blood pressure medications known as ACE inhibitors should be particularly alert for hypoglycemia. A researcher at the Ninewells Hospital in Dundee, Scotland, analyzed hospital admissions for hypoglycemia and ACE inhibitors, a type of blood pressure medication. He found people using the blood pressure medications were three times more likely to be hospitalized with severe hypoglycemia than those who did not take the drugs.

If you use ACE inhibitors to manage your high blood pressure, talk with your health care team about how to limit your hypoglycemia risk. Never stop taking your high blood pressure medication without first talking with your health care team, as hypertension also can be a complication of diabetes that contributes to other diabetes-related conditions.

Treatment. Because your body's use of insulin is determined by many factors, such as stress, exercise, the kinds of food you eat, when you eat it and how much, and the overall state of your health, monitor your blood glucose levels carefully and frequently. Be alert for symptoms that can vary, and take action immediately by eating or drinking a sugar that can enter your digestion and bloodstream quickly. Possibilities include glucose pills or gels. Don't use candy or chocolate, as the fat in these can slow sugar absorption.

Then retest your blood glucose levels about fifteen minutes later. You may need to add another small dose of sugar, but take care to avoid a too-rapid rise in blood glucose that can occur from too much sugar.

After repeated bouts of hypoglycemia, some people lose the ability to detect when one is coming on; others have difficulty detecting it, even with tight control. Protect yourself by eliciting the help of family, friends, and coworkers. Educate them about the symptoms, including the possibility of anger and out-of-control behavior, and the appropriate actions to take. Make clear that hypoglycemia is a life-threatening condition and that if they are unable to intervene, the next step is to call for emergency medical assistance. Your life could be in their hands.

Hypoglycemia at night is a problem that can be particularly perplexing for people with diabetes. Traditionally, treatment has included having a snack before bed to prevent low glucose levels during the night. At Washington University School of Medicine, researchers studied fifteen people with type 1 diabetes and found that when taken at bedtime, alanine, an amino acid, stimulated release of glucagon, while terbutaline normalized blood glucose. Thus, these medications may be a way to avoid hypoglycemia at night.

Hyperglycemia

Hyperglycemic hyperosmolar nonketotic syndrome (HHNS) is most common in people with type 2 diabetes, especially those who do not use insulin. Symptoms include:

- Extreme thirst and a parched mouth.
- Confusion or sleepiness.
- Dry skin, inability to perspire.
- Blurred vision.
- Hunger.
- Nausea.
- Frequent urination.
- Extremely high blood glucose levels.

HHNS occurs when blood glucose levels continually increase. Urine output speeds up; as a result, you become dehydrated. Over time—sometimes days or even weeks—you may become confused and unable to ask for water or to make it to the bathroom. As the blood becomes thicker due to the glucose buildup and dehydration, you may have seizures, go into a coma, and even die.

Treatment. Drink plenty of alcohol-free liquids throughout the day. Checking your blood glucose levels once a day can alert you to impending HHNS. If your level is greater than 350 mg/dl, call your health care team; greater than 500 mg/dl, go immediately to the hospital. People who also take medications such as steroids, diuretics, Dilantin, Tagamet, or beta blockers may need to test their blood glucose more often.

HHNS is especially a risk for people who receive intravenous feedings or peritoneal dialysis. About one-third of HHNS occurs in people in nursing homes who become dehydrated because they must wait for staff to provide liquids. Frequent blood glucose monitoring is the best solution.

●●

BOX 9.1

AN ASPIRIN A DAY KEEPS THE DOCTOR AWAY

Diabetes carries a two to four times higher risk for early death from heart disease.

The ADA recommends that 81 mg to 325 mg of enteric-coated aspirin be used:

Secondary Prevention:

Patients with large vessel disease

Primary Prevention:

Patients with the following risks:

High blood pressure
Obesity
High urine protein
Cigarette smokers
Total cholesterol greater than 200 mg/dL
LDL cholesterol greater than 130 mg/dL
HDL cholesterol less than 40 mg/dL
Triglycerides greater than 250 mg/dL

●●

Cardiovascular Complications

If you have diabetes, you're two to four times more likely to develop cardiovascular disease and five times more likely to have a stroke than those without diabetes. More than half the deaths in people with diabetes are due to heart disease.

It all comes down to blood flow. Blood transports oxygen, glucose, nutrients, and other essential substances to the tissues of the body. If that flow is interrupted or slowed due to uncontrolled blood glucose levels, tissues and vital organs suffer and even may die.

Atherosclerosis. Unchecked blood glucose levels change the chemistry of the bloodstream. Those changes can lead to the clogging of vessels. This clogging may be the result of too many lipids—cholesterol and triglycerides—in the blood.

This buildup can cause these substances to cling to the sides of veins and arteries, narrowing them. Add to that the stickiness of too much glucose, and the process is accelerated. Platelet changes in the blood due to uncontrolled blood glucose levels also can contribute to vessel narrowing.

Treatment. A low-fat, high-fiber diet that minimizes the fat, cholesterol, and triglycerides in the blood, plus exercise, can make a difference. Medications can help control the buildup of substances that clog the circulatory system.

Treatment with large doses of vitamin E, a potent antioxidant, also may offer help. In a study of twenty-eight people with diabetes at the Center for Human Nutrition at the University of Texas Southwest Medical Center, researchers found 1,200 IUs of vitamin E contributed to a decreased risk of heart attack. At the same time, it also reduced rates of LDL, or so-called bad cholesterol. The study builds on the findings of other research involving people without diabetes, which appeared to show that vitamin E reduces LDL levels by blocking its oxidation.

Before increasing your vitamin E intake from the recommended daily average of 10 milligrams, talk with your health care team to be sure intensive vitamin E supplementation is right for you.

Angina. More commonly known as chest pain, angina occurs when blocked vessels restrict blood flow to and from the heart.

Treatment. Medications that widen vessels and arteries or reduce the buildup of plaque in the bloodstream.

Heart attack. Occurring when blocked vessels to the heart are completely blocked by deposits, heart attack is a significant issue for people with diabetes.

Treatment. Medications that widen vessels and arteries or reduce the buildup of plaque in the bloodstream are the most frequent solutions. In advanced cases, arterial bypass surgery to create new paths for blood flow may be necessary. The bypass itself is created by removing vessels from another part of the body, usually the legs, and using them to create new routes for blood flow to and from the heart.

People with diabetes heal more slowly than those without the disease and have higher rates of infection, both of which can be serious postsurgical complications.

High blood pressure. Nearly 60 percent of people with type 2 diabetes have high blood pressure. Hypertension means your heart has to work harder to move blood to and from the heart; that extra work can damage the circulatory system. Eventually, due to the buildup of atheroma—fatty tissue—veins and arteries may be completely blocked.

Treatment. Maintain your weight in a normal range and eat a low-fat, low-sodium diet; with your doctor's approval, exercise twenty to thirty minutes three to four times a week or more. Above all, stop smoking. All of these can help lower blood pressure.

Medications also are available to lower blood pressure, as well as to reduce blood clotting and lower cholesterol. Surgical interventions may include balloon angioplasty to open blocked vessels and arthrectomy to bore away blockages.

Elevated cholesterol. Diabetes can change the number and makeup of proteins that deliver lipids (fats) to the cells. Elevated cholesterol and blood lipids also can accumulate if you eat too much fat. With too much blood glucose in the bloodstream, lipoproteins become extra sticky.

Treatment. Rigorous blood glucose management and a diet that's low in fat and high in fiber, plus regular, physician-approved exercise, can go a long way toward good cholesterol management. In addition, researchers have found that simvastatin, one of the new classes of cholesterol-lowering drugs, can significantly lower cholesterol levels and dramatically reduce heart attack risk.

In one European study, 202 people with diabetes were part of a 4,444-person study of the drug. Results indicated that simvastatin appeared to reduce LDLs, increase HDLs, and lower cholesterol; people with diabetes benefited the most.

Simvastatin lowered their risk of heart attack by 55 percent, compared with 32 percent among persons without diabetes. Additionally, the death rate from heart attack among participants with diabetes dropped to 43 percent, compared to 29 percent among people without diabetes. Researchers believe simvastatin also has no effect on blood glucose levels, making it particularly appealing for people with diabetes.

Stroke. Rates of stroke are two to four times higher among people with diabetes than in the general population. Strokes commonly occur when a small chunk of the plaque that has built up on the lining of vessels and arteries breaks free and circulates in the body until it reaches a passageway through which it cannot pass. This blockage can result in a stroke.

 Treatment. Keeping blood pressure under control, eating a low-fat, high-fiber diet, and exercising regularly with your doctor's approval are the best ways to reduce stroke risk. Your physician also may recommend medications to lower blood pressure and dissolve clots. How well you relate to stressful situations also has an effect on stroke risk.

Intermittent claudication (IC). More commonly referred to as leg pain, IC occurs when vessels and arteries in the legs are partially or fully blocked or restricted.

 Treatment. Exercise and stopping smoking are the best preventions. Your doctor also may recommend medications commonly used to treat blocked vessels and arteries as well as surgery to remove blockages.

Dementia. The specter of developing dementia later in life as a result of uncontrolled blood pressure is a complication that has recently gained attention.

Treatment. Keeping blood pressure at or near normal levels through medication, exercise, and diet may help.

Vision

Diabetes is the leading cause of new blindness among adults. Indeed, people with diabetes are four times more likely to become blind than people without the disease.

Diabetic retinopathy. This is the most common cause of blindness among people with diabetes. Retinopathy is caused by damage to the vessels supplying blood to the retina, and most people don't notice it in its early stages. When detected early by your doctor, retinopathy can be successfully treated and additional vision loss prevented. Even so, it is so common among people with diabetes that after fifteen years of the disease, 80 percent of people not using insulin and 97 percent of those using insulin show some signs of retinopathy.

The two major types of retinopathy are nonproliferative, sometimes called background retinopathy, and proliferative retinopathy. In the former, vessels in the eye close off or weaken and leak blood, fluid, and fat into the eye, blurring vision. This blurred vision can cause blindness if the leaking occurs in the area of the retina near the optic nerve.

Less common, proliferative retinopathy occurs when new blood vessels grow in the retina. These new vessels grow differently than the original ones, rupturing easily. These ruptures are especially common if you also have high blood pressure. Following ruptures, blood may leak into the fluid of the eye, blocking the retina and/or forming scar tissue. If the scar tissue shrinks, it can tear the retina.

Treatment. Prevention and early detection are the most effective solutions, so people with diabetes should have their eyes checked annually after age thirty. Working to keep your blood glucose levels at or near normal also can minimize the occurrence of this condition.

A blood pressure drug, lisinopril, recently has been shown to slow the progression of diabetic retinopathy. A British study of 530 people with type 1 diabetes published in *Lancet* found that at the end of the two-year study, those who had received lisinopril had a slower progression of retinopathy as well as lower blood sugar levels.

Laser treatments can be used to burn away abnormal blood vessels, cauterize leaking ones, and impede the development of new vessels. For some people vitrectomy—a procedure that removes the excess blood and scar tissue, stops bleeding, and replaces some of the substances within the eye, while also repairing the damaged retina—can be helpful.

Retinopathy has a tendency to progress during pregnancy, especially if the mother has had diabetes for ten years or more. Laser surgery may be helpful; even so, some vision may be lost.

Glaucoma. Glaucoma is nearly 1.5 times more common among people with diabetes than among those who don't have the disease. It is a condition in which the pressure of the fluid in the eye is so abnormally high that it compresses and obstructs the vessels supplying blood as well as the optic nerve.

Symptoms include dull, severe aching in and above the eye, fogged vision, and perception of rainbow rings around lights. Nausea and vomiting can occur, and the eye can become red and have a partly dilated pupil and a hazy cornea. The most common type—open-angle glaucoma—rarely occurs before age forty; closed-angle glaucoma has a rapid onset caused by a sudden, complete blockage of the outflow of fluid from the eye.

Treatment. Early detection through testing by an eye specialist is the key because the damage done by mounting pressure in the eye can be irreversible. Open-angle glaucoma can be treated with drops, which reduce the pressure in the eye. In more resistant cases, oral medication may be used. A third, more aggressive technique that uses laser surgery to open the drainage channel in the eye or to create an artificial channel may be needed. Closed-angle glaucoma is a medical emergency that demands immediate attention to save vision.

Cataract. Cataracts are 1.6 times more likely among people with diabetes than in those who don't have the disease. Among people with diabetes, they also occur at a younger age and progress much more rapidly. A cataract occurs because of a loss of transparency in the lens of the eye. This loss of transparency, over time, limits visual acuity and causes color perception to be dulled.

Treatment. Eye surgery to replace the clouded lens with a new, artificial one.

Additional diabetes-related vision complications include:

- **Macular edema.** Resulting from obstruction of circulation to the macula, the central portion of the retina, macular edema causes an overall decrease in vision acuity. As a result, swelling occurs and is often accompanied by a hard lipid accumulation in the macular that may form a ring shape.

- **Neovascularization.** Occurring most often in the nonretinal areas of the eye such as the iris, it produces rubeosis iridis. It also may occur in the rear chamber of the eye, causing hemorrhagic glaucoma.

Nephropathy

After fifteen years of having diabetes, 10 to 20 percent of people with type 2 diabetes develop kidney disease. Diabetes is the leading cause of end-stage renal disease or kidney failure, accounting for about 40 percent of new cases. Research at the University of Minnesota and Northwestern University Medical School found in a study of 332,544 men between thirty-five and fifty-seven that those with diabetes were at thirteen times greater risk for advanced kidney failure.

Dietary changes may provide some answers. At the New England Medical Center in Boston, a review of five studies comparing people with low-protein diets with those who ate average amounts found that those on the low-protein diet had slower rates of kidney disease.

This finding assessed the low-protein diet as leading to a 44 percent reduced risk for diabetic kidney disease and may hold cues for preventing this kidney failure. Before changing your diet, talk with your health care team to be sure a low-protein diet, including cutting back on meat, dairy products, nuts, and beans while eating mostly fruit, vegetables, and grains, is right for you.

Acute renal failure. In end-stage renal disease, the kidneys fail to clear the blood of waste and toxins, so the patient goes into acute renal failure and depends on frequent kidney dialysis to survive. In 1995 nearly 28,000 people with diabetes developed end-stage renal disease.

Treatment. Almost 100,000 people with diabetes were undergoing dialysis or received kidney transplants in 1995. During pregnancy, renal complications may increase for the mother. The amount of protein spilled into the urine during pregnancy should be rigorously monitored. Bed rest is the best treatment; medications also may be necessary.

Neuropathy

The connection between diabetes and damage to the nervous system is clear, but not totally explained. While complications from diabetes generally do not impair the brain or spinal cord, they can alter, damage dramatically, and even destroy other nervous system functions.

About 60 to 70 percent of people with diabetes have mild to severe forms of nervous system damage ranging from loss of sensation in the hands and feet to impaired digestion and other complications. In its most severe form, disease can lead to amputation: More than half the lower limb amputations in the United States occur among people with diabetes.

Distal symmetric polyneuropathy (DSP). This condition can attack the nerves of disparate parts of the body. As a result, arms, hands, legs, and/or feet may feel numb, have no sensitivity to heat and cold, or have sharp stabbing pains or a "pins and needles" sensation; you may not have an awareness of the position of these body parts.

Treatment. Rigorous blood glucose control can help these symptoms disappear, although it may take as long as a year. Therapeutic exercise and the use of some medications can help, as can the topical application of over-the-counter products containing capsaicin, an extract of hot peppers.

A new study in Sweden involving 126 adults with diabetes and neuropathy found that Mexiletine, a drug commonly prescribed to steady irregular heartbeats, may relieve nerve pain. Study participants who received Mexiletine reported significantly less pain and also that they were able to sleep better as a result of less pain.

Focal neuropathy. Less common than DSP, focal neuropathy occurs as a result of damage to a single nerve or group of nerves. In general, it can cause symptoms such as tingling, burning, and numbness. Carpal tunnel syndrome is a typical example. It occurs when the median nerve of the forearm is squeezed by the carpal bones of the wrist.

Treatment. Once good blood glucose control is achieved, symptoms usually disappear.

Autonomic neuropathy. Since the autonomic nervous system controls involuntary activities of the body—digestion, sexual response, sweating—it can be particularly perplexing. Damage to the autonomic nervous system can have disparate and challenging results for people with type 2 diabetes.

Gastrointestinal upset. Ranging from nausea and vomiting to constipation and diarrhea, this diabetes complication can slow the action of the stomach or gut muscles. That slowing can lead to inefficient emptying of the digestive tract.

Treatment. Changes in eating habits such as smaller meals or more frequent meals or just eating soft or liquid foods may help. With the help of your health care team you may need to experiment to find a diet that will work for you. Medications can help to promote stomach emptying and minimize constipation and diarrhea.

Diabetic gastroparesis. Occurring because the stomach empties slowly, diabetic gastroparesis is caused by damage to the nerves that control the pace at which food leaves the stomach and is digested. Symptoms include nausea and/or a sensation of fullness. The result for people with diabetes is that if food empties slowly and you have taken insulin before the meal, blood sugar may fall before the food has had a chance to be absorbed. Diets high in fat and fiber tend to worsen gastroparesis.

Treatment. Work with your health care team to find a solution that's right for you. You may need to take insulin right at the start of a meal to prevent low blood sugars and to match carbohydrate absorption. Medication also may be used to speed digestion.

Incontinence. When nerves to the bladder are damaged, muscles may become weak. As a result, bladder distention, leaking, or difficulty emptying the bladder may occur.

Treatment. Bladder control training, in which the bladder is emptied on a regular schedule, can help. Some people find applying external pressure to the bladder aids in completely emptying the bladder, which can forestall leakage. Men may find it helpful to urinate seated. Medication, a catheter, or surgery are other alternatives.

Loss of sexual function or desire. Sexual function is a complex topic. For instance, sexual arousal for men and women is essentially a function of the autonomic nervous system. Yet the ability to engage in and enjoy intercourse is a complicated marriage of mental, emotional, and physical capabilities.

For people with diabetes, this intricate process is increased by the impact complications can have on the various systems and responses that make sexual activity possible and enjoyable. Men with diabetes develop impotence ten to fifteen years earlier than those without the disease; 50 to 60 percent of all men over fifty who have diabetes also have some problems with impotence.

Some 35 percent of women with diabetes experience some level of diminished sexual function, including reduced sensitivity to touch due to nerve damage as well as poor bladder control, vaginal dryness, or lessened sexual desire.

The pressures of managing diabetes and the fear of experiencing hypoglycemia after intercourse can be a damper on a lovemaking session. So, too, can the loss of self-esteem that diabetes and its complications bring, such as amputations, infection, incontinence, and slow-healing injuries.

Treatment. Keeping blood glucose levels as close to normal as possible is important in preserving your ability to enjoy and engage in sexual activities. If you are experiencing sexual difficulties, talk with your health care team about suggestions and solutions. Don't assume you have to learn to live with this complication.

For women, lost sensitivity may be addressed with changes in sexual technique, a more gentle or creative approach on the part of the partner. Vaginal dryness may be due to hormonal issues that may or may not be related to diabetes. Talk with your gynecologist about hormonal testing to ensure your levels are where they should be. Your gynecologist may suggest hormone replacement therapy or over-the-counter lubricants. Poor bladder control may be resolved by emptying your bladder thirty minutes before sex. This has the added benefit of reducing occurrence of bladder infections. Women with diabetes frequently experience vaginal candida infections. The chances of this happening can be lessened by using a small amount of antifungal cream as a lubricant. Boston University is studying whether the new medication for impotence, Viagra, may help women reclaim their sexuality.

Impotence in men may be the result of blood vessel damage or nerve disease. A urologist can help diagnose the specific cause and recommend medication, therapies, or surgeries that can restore full or partial function. New medications, such as Viagra, as well as Vasomax and apomorphine, may be appropriate for some men.

Men can help preserve their ability to perform sexually by quitting smoking, decreasing alcohol intake, and exercising regularly.

Some medications for high blood pressure control can contribute to impotence, as can drugs for depression, anxiety, and peptic ulcers. If you use these medications, talk with your doctor about changes in dosage or other approaches to reduce their interference with sexual performance. Never stop taking medications without first talking with your doctor.

Postural dizziness. When you exercise, you may find your blood pressure rises quickly: Rising from a seated position or standing for long periods may leave you feeling light-headed or dizzy.

Treatment. This complication seems to be related to damage to the heart and blood vessels. If you drink alcohol, that, too, can cause blood pressure variations. Such medications as antidepressants, diuretics, nitroglycerin, and some calcium-blocking drugs also can contribute. If you take these, talk with your health care team about ways in which dosages may be adjusted to minimize their effect on postural dizziness.

Other strategies your health care team may recommend include medication for low blood pressure or taking a proactive approach, such as rising from a seated position slowly or avoiding standing for long periods of time. Wearing support stockings to prevent blood from pooling in your legs may also be a solution. If postural dizziness occurs most often upon rising from bed, try raising the head of the bed six to nine inches. This slight elevation may help bridge the gap from being in a prone position to standing.

Gustatory sweating. While eating, some people with diabetes break out in a sweat or experience flushing of the neck and chest.

Treatment. The exact cause of gustatory sweating isn't known, but it's believed to be related to having had high blood glucose levels for long periods of time. It appears to be brought on by eating cheese or chocolate, as well as salty foods such as pickles, alcohol, fresh fruit, and vinegar, so avoiding these also may limit or eliminate gustatory sweating. Significant improvement can be achieved by keeping your blood glucose levels in check.

Your health care team may recommend medications. One medication developed in the United Kingdom contains glycopyrrolate. British doctors tested a cream containing this substance on thirteen people with diabetes. After using the cream, test subjects found sweating was stopped or significantly reduced.

Charcot's joints. Most often affecting weight-bearing joints such as ankles, Charcot's usually starts with bone thinning and a loss of feeling, especially in the extremities. Since bones are weakened and feeling absent, breaks may occur, but go unnoticed, despite swelling. (Charcot's is sometimes misdiagnosed as osteoarthritis [OA], but Charcot's progresses much more rapidly than OA.) Because there's little or no pain due to neuropathy, you continue to use the affected joint. The injury worsens, muscles shrink, and the joint may become deformed.

Treatment. Good blood glucose control can help prevent this condition. Early diagnosis is key in alleviating serious, permanent injury to joints. Treatment may include use of splints to prevent additional joint deformity.

Foot drop. This is condition in which the foot cannot be raised properly due to damage to the nerves that supply the foot. The foot hangs limply from the ankle joint, causing it to catch as you walk.

    Treatment. Your physician may recommend a wearing a splint, brace, or other support to keep the foot in a proper position for walking.

Finger stiffness. Because of high blood sugar over long periods of time, the tissue around the joints of your fingers may become stiff. This stiffness can keep you from straightening your fingers and make it hard for you to write, dress yourself, tie your shoes, or pick up small objects.

    To test yourself for this, hold your hands together with the palms facing and pressing together. If there's space between your right and left hands, you may have "positive prayer sign," another diabetes complication.

    Treatment. Keeping your blood glucose levels at or near normal is the best treatment.

Memory loss. Poor blood glucose control appears to contribute to memory loss. An analysis of nineteen diabetes studies seems to indicate loss of memory and other cognitive function may be related to diabetes. The ability to remember words appears to be the most affected.

    Treatment. Good blood glucose control appears to be the most effective treatment in preserving memory.

Other diabetic neuropathic conditions include:

- Muscle wasting (atrophy) and paralysis as the result of nerve damage.
- Paralysis of eye muscles so the eyes no longer track in unison.
- Hammer toes, named for the distinctive, hammer-shaped position the toes take on. This complication occurs due to changes in muscle or in bony structures. It exposes the metatarsal heads of the feet, creating a greater potential for trauma and ulcer formation.
- Rocker foot, which occurs as bony structures continue to change and a loss of sensation in the ankle leads to a relaxation of supporting tissues. The ankle becomes inflamed and the foot shortens and widens while the arch flattens.

Dental

Aggressive periodontal disease, gum-line cavities, dry mouth and infection are common among people with type 2 diabetes.

Treatment. Combined with rigorous blood glucose control, energetic daily dental hygiene can help prevent or minimize dental complications for patients with type 2 diabetes. You also should see your dentist twice a year for regular exams and cleanings to prevent plaque buildup, which can increase the likelihood of gum disease.

Protect your teeth and gums with good glucose control plus these dental hygiene basics.

- Brush your teeth twice a day with a soft nylon brush that has rounded ends on the bristles. Also brush the rough upper surface of your tongue.
- Floss daily.

Call your dentist if:

- Your gums are red, swollen, or tender; bleed when you brush your teeth; or appear to be pulling away from your teeth.
- You find pus between your teeth and gums when you touch the gums.
- The fit of your dentures or partial plate changes or your bite changes.
- You have a persistent bad taste in your mouth or bad breath.
- You have a consistent sore or "raw" throat.

Infection

Type 2 diabetes can put you at risk for a wide variety of infections. That's because an excess of glucose makes immune cells less effective. And many infection-causing agents—bacteria, viruses, and fungi—feed on the excess glucose.

Damaged nerves and reduced circulation can further complicate and increase the risk of infection. In the absence of feeling, injuries may go unnoticed, creating opportunities for infection to set in and progress without immediate detection. Reduced circulation means people with diabetes take longer than people who don't have diabetes to heal from injuries, whether the injury is an ingrown toenail or a major surgical incision.

Urinary tract infections. Because of damage to the nerves, incomplete bladder emptying may occur. This unemptied urine is fertile ground for bacteria growth, resulting in frequent bladder infections.

Treatment. Emptying the bladder on a regular schedule and using external pressure to facilitate emptying can help. If bladder infections persist, your health care team may recommend antibiotics or solutions such as a catheter.

Vaginal yeast infections. The yeast, *Candida albicans,* which naturally inhabits a woman's vaginal tract, thrives where the environment is moist and glucose is abundant. It's a combination of conditions some women with diabetes provide.

Treatment. While a yeast infection can be very uncomfortable, with burning and itching that may be accompanied by a white discharge, it's usually not a danger to your health. To reduce the chances of developing a yeast infection:

- Wear breathable, all-cotton underwear and change it daily.
- Avoid pantyhose and pants that are tight and restrict air flow.

Your gynecologist can recommend medications to relieve symptoms and eliminate the infection. The best long-term solution is good blood glucose control.

Foot ulcers and ulcerations. More likely to occur when circulation to the foot is poor and blood glucose levels uncontrolled, foot ulcers and ulcerations occur when a minor injury goes untreated. Infections set in, rapidly destroying layers of skin and other tissues and even reaching and infecting the bone.

Indiana University School of Medicine researchers found in a study of 352 people with type 2 diabetes that foot ulcers were most common among those over forty who also were overweight and had neuropathy in their legs, with an inability to sense temperature changes. Other predictors include:

Dry and/or cracked foot skin.
Poorly trimmed toenails.
Fungal foot and nail infections.

Treatment. Good blood glucose control and diligent foot care are still the best ways to prevent foot ulcers. At the same time, physicians recently have determined that treating ulcers with collagen may facilitate healing. In shallow ulcers, the collagen is applied topically. In deep ulcers, the wound must first be cleared surgically of dead and dying tissue, usually under local anesthetic. Then collagen, and antibiotics to control infection, are packed into the wound.

Other foot ulcer treatments showing promise are:

- Dermagraft, a bioabsorbable mesh onto which special skin cells from newborns have been added.

- Regranex, a gel that promises to speed the healing of foot ulcers by 43 percent when applied once a day.

- Electric stimulation that activates the nerves and increases the blood flow.

In extreme cases, surgery may be necessary to remove the infected area; amputation is a possibility.

Gangrene. An advanced stage of infection, gangrene means affected tissues have died, usually as the result of infection or lost blood supply. This is a serious medical emergency that can occur when a person with diabetes fails to seek proper care for an injury.

Treatment. Without proper medical care, usually antibiotics and surgical removal of affected tissues, a gangrene infection can spread to invade other tissues. In some cases, amputation is the only way to remove diseased tissue and save the patient's life.

Staphylococcal infections. These occur as itchy spots on the buttocks, knees, and elbows.

BOX 9.2

PREVENTION OF AMPUTATIONS

- 67,000 lower limbs are lost yearly in the United States to diabetes-related problems; greater than half of these losses could be prevented with early detection and treatment.
- The amputation rate for blacks is 1.5 to 2.5 times greater than whites.
- The amputation rate for Native Americans is 3 to 4 times higher than the general population.

The American Podiatric Medical Association is teaching people how to prevent diabetic related amputations. The toll-free number is 1-800-615-0807 or their Web site is www.apma.org.

Treatment. See your doctor, who may recommend topical treatment to eliminate the infection and relieve symptoms.

Good foot care. If you have diabetes, restricted circulation and nerve damage can make your feet vulnerable to a wide variety of conditions and to injuries. The injured feet of a person with diabetes heal slowly, and that creates a window for infection. To limit damage and injury to your feet remember:

- Inspect your feet daily for blisters, cuts, scratches, and tenderness. If necessary, use a mirror to examine thoroughly the underside of feet.
- Wash your feet thoroughly at least once a day. Dry carefully and completely between the toes.
- Inspect the insides of shoes daily for objects and torn or rough areas; be sure your shoes contain plenty of room in the toe box and fit comfortably in the heel. Consider having your shoes custom-fitted.
- Wear only shoes made of breathable materials, and change shoes at least daily.
- Avoid temperature extremes by testing bathwater before stepping in.
- Use lotion on your feet but avoid getting it between the toes; your health care team may recommend over-the-counter or prescription lotions to ease dryness and callus buildup.
- Do not use heating pads or hot water bottles, and avoid soaking your feet in hot water.
- Cut nails in contour with the toes; better yet, have them trimmed by a podiatrist.

- Don't use chemical plasters or ointment to remove corns or calluses; do not cut corns or calluses away.

- Do not use adhesive tape, as it can irritate the skin.

- Never walk barefoot or wear open-toed shoes.

- If your feet have decreased sensation, break in shoes slowly, wearing different pairs throughout the day.

- Notify your doctor immediately if you find a blister, crack, cut, or other inflammation on your feet.

Mental Health

Living with diabetes can be stressful. For people with diabetes, everyday decisions can be crucial ones of continued well-being and long-term health. While the occurrence of depression is the same for people with and without diabetes, people with diabetes may find themselves grappling with depression for reasons that are specific to their disease.

The links between depression and diabetes generally relate to concerns about:

- Long-term physical health.

- Financial demands of diabetes, as well as barriers the disease may present to work.

- Changes in relationships with family and friends, employer, and activities you love best as a result of coping with diabetes.

Depending on your ability to control your disease, you may be fearful of hypoglycemia or hyperglycemia. You may feel anxious about managing medication correctly. And if you already are experiencing complications such as retinopathy or sexual dysfunction, anxiety may increase exponentially.

If you're seriously depressed, the distress can actually alter your ability to manage your blood glucose levels. And it can contribute to such behaviors as inappropriate diet, alcohol use, and failure to exercise. Depression can intensify discomfort you may be feeling as a result of other complications.

Treatment. Talking with your health care team can help you gain confidence and the knowledge you need to manage your disease successfully. That confidence, when combined with the help of a support group, may aid you in achieving more stable and hopeful feelings about your life.

Exercise can be especially helpful in relieving symptoms of depression and anxiety. That's good news because regular, physician-approved exercise can play a key role in diabetes management, weight loss, and reduction of complications.

An Indiana University study found that just twenty minutes of leg exercises led to a drop in anxiety levels, even when the exercises were done in a mild way and at a light pace. The researchers further found that just five minutes of exercise led to a reduction in anxiety levels that could still be felt two hours later. They speculate that longer, more intense exercise sessions could have greater benefits.

Medication and therapy also may be options. Three studies in the 1997 issue of *Psychological Annals, Psychosomatic Medicine and Diabetes* have shown that people with diabetes respond equally well to antidepressant medication and to therapy.

Symptoms of Depression. If you experience three or more of the following symptoms for two weeks or longer, or if you are having suicidal thoughts, seek help from a mental health professional.

- Feelings of sadness, hopelessness, and extreme irritability.
- Loss of interest or pleasure from activities you previously enjoyed.
- Trouble sleeping, sleeping too much, or awakening at an inappropriate time and being unable to go back to sleep.
- Weight loss or weight gain.
- Difficulty concentrating.
- Extreme tiredness or loss of energy.
- Anxious feelings or guilt.

Pancreatic Cancer

Researchers at the National Institutes of Diabetes and Digestive and Kidney Diseases (NIDDK) have reported a finding that may indicate a connection between diabetes and pancreatic cancer.

NIDDK researchers reported this potential connection based on review of twenty studies done between 1975 and 1994 that dealt with pancreatic cancer risk factors. In eighteen of the twenty, diabetes emerged as a risk factor.

Treatment. Good blood glucose control and a healthy lifestyle remain the strongest lines of defense against diabetic complications.

Pregnancy and Diabetes Complications

Whether you had diabetes before you became pregnant or developed gestational diabetes, staying healthy and having a healthy baby present particular challenges to women with diabetes.

Women with diabetes who want to become pregnant should talk with their health care team about the steps they can take to minimize complications. For a woman whose pregnancy precedes her diabetes, there are many challenges.

The pregnant woman with diabetes who already has complications may find that the severity of these increases and must manage all aspects of her disease rigorously during pregnancy. In some cases, your doctor may recommend avoiding pregnancy because it could put your health at risk, particularly if you already have cardiovascular disease, kidney failure, or serious gastrointestinal neuropathy.

The pregnant woman with diabetes is at increased risk for high blood pressure.

Birth defects are another complication whose potential should be carefully assessed before pregnancy. The average risk of birth defects is 2 to 3 percent for healthy women; for babies whose mothers have diabetes and maintain good blood glucose control, the risk is 6 to 12 percent. Typical defects include central nervous system abnormalities as well as heart and kidney defects.

Gestational diabetes. Gestational diabetes is a usually temporary form of diabetes that occurs when the hormones associated with pregnancy create extra insulin resistance. It's most often identified about halfway through pregnancy. Risk factors for gestational diabetes include:

- A family history of diabetes.
- A history of gestational diabetes in previous pregnancies.
- A history of glucose intolerance outside of pregnancy.
- Obesity.
- Patient's own birth weight greater than nine pounds.
- Poor obstetrics history, for example, habitual abortions or a previous baby with a birth weight greater than nine pounds.
- Unexplained stillbirths.
- Birth defects in other children.
- History of toxemia.
- Recurrent urinary tract infections.
- Excess amniotic fluid.

Being overweight appears to be a significant contributing factor; a pregnant woman who is overweight has a three in four chance of developing gestational diabetes.

True gestational diabetes disappears after delivery. Women who have had gestational diabetes are at greater risk for developing type 2 diabetes five to fifteen years after pregnancy. A small number of women continue to have diabetes after delivery. They are generally believed to be people who were previously undiagnosed and whose disease was made evident by pregnancy.

BOX 9.3

RECOMMENDATIONS FOR CARE
OF TYPE-2 DIABETES

Yearly (in addition to the quarterly recommendations)

Complete physical examination.

Complete eye examination, with dilitation by an ophthalmologist.

Blood chemistry analysis with a fasting lipid profile.

Urinary testing for microalbuminuria.

If cardiac disease present—electrocardiogram.

Quarterly

Blood pressure check, pulse, heart rate.

Foot examination by a podiatrist.

HbA1c (glycohemoglobin) measurement and evaluation.

Review of self glucose monitoring (SGB) results.

Monthly

Self-review of dietary management.

Glycoprotein analysis (fructosamine testing).

Feet inspection for sores, cracks, potential problems.

Urinary testing for protein.

Review of lifestyle goals.

Modification of diabetes cure plan if needed.

Finally, the Good News

Just knowing about the complications of diabetes can be depressing. Diabetes at its worst is among the most devastating of all diseases, namely because it has the ability to exploit a person's physical weaknesses, no matter what they are.

How could there possibly be any good news about diabetes?

Well, there is, and it is this: Type 2 diabetes is a disease of lifestyle that can be reversed by adopting healthy habits. You don't have to be a victim of this terrible disease if you take control and decide you are going to beat it.

Yes, diabetes is beatable, and with this book you have the tools to do just that. As I tell my patients, "I can give you the road map to get to wellness, but you have to drive the car."

Drive carefully.

10

The Future Is Now

The discovery in 1921 that the injection of secretions from a portion of the pancreas—islets of Langerhans—could relieve symptoms of diabetes changed lives. Since then, research has developed new techniques and treatments that improve the lives of people with diabetes even as understanding of the mechanisms and side effects of type 2 diabetes continue to emerge.

Despite all the new and improved methods of treating type 2 diabetes, prevention still stands out as the single most effective way to avoid or limit diabetic complications. For those who have type 2 diabetes, self-monitoring and serious attention to lifestyle changes still stand as the best ways to control, slow, and even reverse the course of diabetes. Most cases of type 2 diabetes can be cured, but it takes serious attention to all aspects of lifestyle that caused the diabetes to begin with. By following the nine steps outlined in the Diabetes Cure, you are doing just that, attacking this insidious disease on all fronts.

The essential role of prevention and self-monitoring was crystallized via the Diabetes Control and Complications Trial (DCCT). Completed in 1993, this nationwide study confirmed that the risk of diabetic complications could be reduced with tight control, keeping blood glucose levels as close to normal as possible. This study confirmed what many had previously thought and further reinforced the role prevention and individual responsibility play in living a long and fulfilling life, despite diabetes. At the same time, results from the DCCT continue to play a part in the development of individualized approaches to diabetes management.

Beyond Prevention

The number of people with type 2 diabetes has risen 700 percent since the 1950s. This increase reflects a number of emerging trends, including the increase in average age of Americans—the most common age at which diabetes is diagnosed is fifty-one.

Other factors include growth among the ethnic populations who appear to be at higher risk for diabetes, as well as increases in weight and decreases in levels of activity across the population. These trends have led to the development and exploration of new and diverse treatments.

Medication

In the past ten years a number of new medications have emerged. In addition to using HCA and following the steps outlined in the Diabetes Cure, you might want to discuss some of these medications with your physician. This is especially true if you are insulin-dependent. *Family Practice News* in 1996 reported that the use of a combination of drugs to treat people with insulin-dependent type 2 diabetes leads to reduced side effects and fewer long-term complications than a single drug. These drugs include:

- The blood pressure drug lisinopril slows the development of diabetic retinopathy, which occurs in 70 percent of people with type 2 diabetes.

- The cholesterol-lowering drug simvastatin is in the newest class of medications for this purpose. In a Swedish study reported in *Diabetes Care*, people with diabetes who used simvastatin experienced a 55 percent decrease in their risk of heart attack.

- The ACE inhibitor fosinopril appears to create a 50 percent lowered risk of stroke, heart attack, and chest pain among people with diabetes and high blood pressure who use the drug.

- Silenafil has been found instrumental for men with diabetes who experience erectile dysfunction as a result of their disease.

- Mexiletine, a cardiac drug with a long history, is now being studied for use in treating people with diabetes who have a painful nerve disease as a result of their condition.

- Tagamet, a medication available since the early 1980s for ulcers and heartburn, is showing promise for people with type 2 diabetes. Researchers at the University of Oslo in Norway found that Tagamet given in a liquid form helped test subjects shed weight, lower blood pressure, and control blood glucose levels.

Tests

- Diabetic kidney disease is the leading cause of people undergoing kidney dialysis. A new test has been developed that detects kidney disease early, allowing for earlier detection and treatment. In combination with ACE inhibitors, this early detection can limit the occurrence of kidney disease, reducing the need for dialysis.

- A test that allows people with diabetes to determine the HbA1c values at home is new to the marketplace. The first of its kind, it allows HbA1c testing with a simple finger prick. The blood sample is then mailed to a lab in a prepaid envelope; results are available in seven to ten days. The availability of this test has changed the lives of many people with diabetes.

BOX 10.1

NO-BLOOD BLOOD TEST??

LifeGuide is the name of a no-blood blood glucose monitor.

Integ, the manufacturer, states the hand-held unit uses a small hollow needle that punctures just underneath the skin and samples the tissue fluid there. This fluid is analyzed by light rays or infared spectroscopy to determine the glucose level. The "bloodless" test is sampled from the forearm rather than the finger as with most units on the market today. This area is less sensitive and should cause less discomfort according to the manufacturer of the device.

For more information visit their Web site at: www.integonline.com.

Other Innovations

Although the Diabetes Cure is essentially a low-technology approach to the control and cure of diabetes, technology does play an important role in monitoring blood glucose. As important as this monitoring is, repeated finger pricks to check glucose levels is one of the frustrations of diabetes. The Food and Drug Administration recently gave approval for sales of the Laser Lancet. It's a small, hand-held battery-powered device that draws blood by sending a brief pulse of highly concentrated laser light through a disposable tube. The light cuts the skin just deep enough to draw blood, but not as deeply as lancets go. Developed by Venise Inc., the device is available only by prescription.

Although the goal of *The Diabetes Cure* is to cure diabetes or lessen its effects, there are people with type 2 diabetes who are using insulin and are frustrated at having to use needle and syringe to administer it. For them, a method of needle-free insulin administration is in development. Sometimes called "the Holy Grail" of diabetes care, it allows people with diabetes to inhale insulin via microscopic particles of crystallized insulin placed inside a plastic tube. Once the particle pack opens, the vapor can be inhaled in one breath. The insulin is absorbed instantly into the bloodstream through the vast surface of the lungs.

Preliminary research is under way in the development of an artificial pancreas. Unlike the insulin pump, which is worn on the outside of the body and the use of which is generally limited to people with type 1 diabetes, this device would be implanted inside the body. It would include the insertion of an internal catheter into the abdominal cavity to convey insulin, plus a built-in glucose sensor and sensitive systems that would automatically detect when the body needs more insulin and automatically release it.

It is good to know about these technological advances, but frankly, I hope you never have to use them. Diabetes can be beaten, and *The Diabetes Cure* provides all of the necessary ingredients for success.

When patients ask me about future medical developments, hoping that a future diabetes medication will have no side effects and will allow them to live their lives unchanged, I tell them that the future is now.

"Without diligent change on your part, modern medicine can only slow the progress of your disease. It cannot cure it," I tell my patients.

If they seem depressed by this information, I tell them about one of my worse-off patients, maybe someone like Maxine.

Maxine illustrates a severe case of type 2 diabetes. Maxine had been placed on insulin for her diabetes about two years prior to seeing me. She had moved to the area recently and was establishing new relationships and finding a new doctor, dentist, and drugstore.

The move was emotionally trying and had left her feeling depressed and fatigued. She felt that her Prozac was not helping her as it used to, and she was frustrated with herself for the short temper she was exhibiting toward her family. Store-bought cookies seemed to help with some of her anxiety, but only temporarily. Maxine wanted help.

Her glucose was "out of control" at 305. Never had it been so consistently high. She had tried several times to lose weight during the past two months, but her scale fluctuated just a few pounds. Determined to get back on track, she began using HCA in addition to the insulin. She noticed that the HCA curbed her appetite, and she felt fuller, faster. Her weight began to drop. After eight weeks, she had lost more than ten pounds. Her fasting glucose dropped with her weight, down to 211. With the drop in weight and the glucose level came a rise in energy.

With a more stable glucose level and body weight, Maxine began to question her endocrinologist about what she needed to do to "get off the insulin." He assured her that if she continued to increase her activity, lose weight, and take HCA with chromium, she would be on the road to stopping her need for insulin altogether.

She commented to her physician, "The Prozac seems to be working better," and acknowledged that all of her was working better. She reported less frustration, less irritability, and more patience in her new surroundings.

Although still seriously overweight, Maxine had realized the importance of focusing on her health. She has now become an advocate for "making time for health," and as a result has more time and energy for other things.

You have in your hands the same guidebook that Maxine and others have used. It is one that can lead you out of the dangerous terrain defined by the disease known as type 2 diabetes. Whether you have diabetes or you are at risk for getting it, now is the time to use the information in this book to put your health in order.

Useful References
•••••••••••••••••••••

Medical Literature

Alterman, Seymour L. *How to Control Diabetes.* New York: Ballantine Books, 1996.

American Diabetes Association. "Clinical Practice Recommendations 1998." Introduction and Position Statement, vol. 21, supplement 1.

Anderson, G. H. "Regulation of Food Intake." In *Modern Nutrition in Health and Disease,* 8th ed., edited by Maurice E. Shils, James A. Olson, and Moshe Shike, pp. 524–536. Philadelphia: Lea and Febiger, 1994.

Barth C., J. Hackenschmidt, H. Ullmann, and K. Decker. "Inhibition of Cholesterol Synthesis by (-)-Hydroxycitrate in Perfused Rat Liver. Evidence for an Extramitochondrial Mevalonate Synthesis from Acetyl Coenzyme A." *Archives of Biochemistry and Biophysics* 22, no. 3 (May 1972): 343–346.

Berkhout, T. A. "The Effect of (-)-Hydroxycitrate on the Activity of the Low-Density-Lipoprotein Receptor and 3-hydroxy–3-methylglutaryl-CoA Reductase Levels in the Human Hepatoma Cell Line Hep G2." *Biochemistry Journal* 272 (1990): 181–186.

Boll, M., E. Sorensen, and E. Balieu. "Naturally Occurring Lactones and Lactames. III. The Absolute Configuration of the Hydroxycitric Acid Lactones: Hibiscus Acid and Garcinia Acid." *Acta Chemica Scandinavica* 23 (1969): 283–293.

Bonadonna, R. C., and R. A. Defronzo. "Glucose Metabolism in Obesity and Type II Diabetes." In *Obesity*, edited by Per Bjorntorp and Bernard N. Brodoff, pp. 474–476. Philadelphia: J. B. Lippincott, 1992.

Bonora, E., C. Coscelli, and U. Butturini. "Relationship Between Insulin Resistance, Insulin Secretion and Insulin Metabolism in Simple Obesity." *International Journal of Obesity* 9 (1985): 307–312.

Bowden, C. R., K. D. White, and G. F. Tutwiler. "Energy Intake of Cafeteria-Diet and Chow-Fed Rats in Response to Amphetamine, Fenfluramine, (-)-Hydroxycitrate, and Naloxone." *Journal of Obesity and Weight Regulation* 4, no. 1 (Spring 1985): 5–13.

Brunengraber, H., J. R. Sabine, M. Boutry, and J. M. Lowenstein. "3-beta-Hydroxysterol Synthesis by the Liver." *Archives of Biochemistry and Biophysics* 150 (1972): 392–396.

Chee, H., D. R. Romsos, and G. A. Leveille. "Influence of (-)-Hydroxycitrate on Lipogenesis in Chickens and Rats." *Journal of Nutrition* 107, no. 1 (1977): 112–119.

Cheema-Dhadli, S., M. L. Halperin, and C. C. Leznoff. "Inhibition of Enzymes Which Interact with Citrate by (-)-Hydroxycitrate and 1,2,3,-Tricarboxybenzene." *European Journal of Biochemistry* 38 (1973): 98–102.

Clouatre, D. *Anti-Fat Nutrients*, 2nd ed. San Francisco: PAX Publishing, 1993.

Clouatre, D., and M. Rosenbaum. "The Diet and Health Benefits of HCA (Hydroxycitric Acid)." New Canaan, Conn.: Keats Publishing, 1994.

Conte, A. A. "A Non-Prescription Alternative in Weight Reduction Therapy." cited in A. Conte and M. Majeed, *A Revolutionary Herbal Approach to Weight Management*, Chapter 6. Burlingame, Calif.: New Editions Publishing, 1994.

Danforth, M. "Weight Loss Clinical Outcome Study." Legere Pharmaceuticals Protocol Using All Natural Agents, June 22, 1998. Abstract, via Legere.

Eastman, R. C. "Prevention of Type 2 Diabetes." *Current Approaches to the Management of Type-2 Diabetes: A Practical Monograph*. National Diabetes Education Initiative for Health Care Professionals, Professional Graduate Services, 1997, pp. 43–46.

Finney, Lois, R. D. Schmidt, and Michael Gonzalez-Campoy. "Dietary Chromium and Diabetes: Is There a Relationship?" *Clinical Diabetes* 15, no. 1 (January–February 1997): 6–8.

Frawley, David. *The Yoga of Herbs*. Santa Fe: Lotus Press, 1986.

Fujimoto, M. D. "A National Multicenter Study to Learn Whether Type II Diabetes Can Be Prevented: The Diabetes Prevention Program." *Clinical Diabetes* 15, no. 1 (January–February 1997): 13–15.

Garber, Alan J. "For Better or for Worse." *Clinical Diabetes* 15, no. 1 (January–February 1997): 2–3.

———. "When Does Diabetes Begin, and How Do We Know It?" *Clinical Diabetes* (July–August 1997): 146–147

Gavin, James R., III, and Hal Singer. "Putting Findings to Work." *Patient Care*, February 15, 1998, pp. 13–14.

Gibbons, G. F. "The Metabolic Route by Which Oleate *is* Converted into Cholesterol in Rat Hepatocytes." *Biochemistry Journal* 235 (1986): 19–24.

Greenwood, M. R. C., M. P. Cleary, R. Gruen, D. Blasé, J. S. Stern, J. Triscari, and A. C. Sullivan. "Effect of (-)-Hydroxycitrate on Development of Obesity in the Zucker Obese Rat." *American Journal of Physiology* 240 (1981): E72–E78.

Guyton, A. C. Chapter 67 in *Textbook of Medical Physiology*, 8th ed. Philadelphia: W. B. Saunders, 1991.

Hirsch, I. B. "Standards of Care for the Treatment of Diabetes." *Clinical Diabetes* 16, no. 1 (1998): 26–29.

Hirsch, J., and R. L. Leibel. "Clinical Review 28: A Biological Basis for Human Obesity." *Journal of Clinical Endocrinology and Metabolism* 73, no. 6 (1991): 1153–1157.

Hobbs, L. S. "(-)-Hydroxycitrate (HCA)." In *The New Diet Pills*, pp. 161–174. Irvine, Calif.: Pragmatic Press, 1994.

Hoffmann, C. E., H. Andres, L. Weiss, C. Kreisel, and R. Sander. "Lipogenesis in Man: Properties and Organ Distribution of ATF Citrate (pro-3S)-Lyase." *Biochimica et Biophysica Acta* 620 (1980): 151–158.

Horton, E. S. "Therapeutic Options for the Treatment of Type 2 Diabetes." *Current Approaches to the Management of Type-2 Diabetes: A Practical Monograph.* National Diabetes Education Initiative for Health Care Professionals, Professional Graduate Services, 1997, pp. 35–42.

Jaedig, S., and N. C. Henningsen. "Increased Metabolic Rate in Obese Women After Ingestion of Potassium, Magnesium- and Phosphate-Enriched Orange Juice or Injection of Ephedrine." *International Journal of Obesity* 15 (1991): 429–436.

Kaats, G. R., D. Pullin, L. K. Parker, P. L. Keith, and S. Keith. "Reductions of Body Fat as a Function of Taking a Dietary Supplement Containing Garcinia Cambogia Extract, Chromium Picolinate and L-Carnitine—A Double Blind Placebo Controlled Study" [abstract]. *Age* 14 (1991): 138.

King, Dana E., Virginia Peragallo-Dittko, William Polonosky, James Proshaska, and Frank Vinicor. "Strategies for Improving Self-Care." *Patient Care*, February 15, 1998, pp. 91–111.

Kitabchi, Abbas E., and Michael Bryer-Ash. "NIDDM: New Aspects of Management." *Hospital Practice*, March 15, 1997, pp. 135–64.

Lean, M. E. "Evidence for Brown Adipose Tissue in Humans." In *Obesity*, edited by Per Bjorntorp and Bernard Brodoff, pp. 117–129. Philadelphia: J. B. Lippincott, 1992.

Leon, Gloria R. "Behavioral Approach to Obesity." *American Journal of Clinical Nutrition* 30 (1977): 785–789.

Levin, B. E., J. Triscari, and A. C. Sullivan. "Altered Sympathetic Activity During Development of Diet-Induced Obesity in Rats." *American Journal of Physiology* 244, no. 2 (1983): R347–R355.

Lewis, Y. S. "Isolation and Properties of Hydroxycitric Acid." In *Citric Acid Cycle*, vol. 13 in *Methods in Enzymology*, edited by John M. Lowenstein, pp. 613–619. New York: Academic Press, 1969.

Lewis, Y. S., and S. Neelakantan. "(-)Hydroxycitric Acid—The Principal Acid in the Fruits of the Garcinia Cambogia." *Phytochemistry* 4 (1965): 619–625.

Lowenstein, J. M. "Effect of (-)-Hydroxycitrate on Fatty Acid Synthesis by Rat Liver in Vivo." *Journal of Biological Chemistry* 246, no. 3 (February 10, 1971): 629–632.

———. "Experiments with (-)-Hydroxycitrate." In *Essays in Cell Metabolism*, edited by W. Bartley, H. L. Kornberg, and J. R. Quayle, pp. 153–166. London: Wiley-Interscience, 1970.

Lowenstein, J. M., and H. Brunengraber. "Hydroxycitrate." In *Lipids*, vol. 72 in *Methods in Enzymology*, edited by John M. Lowenstein, pp. 486–497. New York: Academic Press, 1981.

Manchester, Jill, Alexander V. Skurat, Peter Roach, Stephen D.

Hauschka, and John C. Lawrence, Jr. "Increased Glycogen Accumulation in Transgenic Mice Overexpressing Glycogen Synthase in Skeletal Muscle." *Proceedings of the National Academy of Sciences* 93, no. 20 (1996): 10707–10711.

Mathias, M. M., A. C. Sullivan, and J. C. Hamilton. "Fatty Acid and Cholesterol Synthesis from Specifically Labeled Leucine by Isolated Rat Hepatocytes." *Lipids* 16, no. 10 (1981): 739–743.

McCarty, M. F. "Inhibition of Citrate Lyase May Aid Aerobic Endurance." *Medical Hypotheses* 45 (1995): 247–254.

———. "Optimizing Exercise for Fat Loss." *Medical Hypotheses* 44 (1995): 325–330.

———. "Promotion of Hepatic Lipid Oxidation and Gluconeogenesis as a Strategy for Appetite Control." *Medical Hypotheses* 42 (1994): 215–225.

———. "Reduction of Free Fatty Acids May Ameliorate Risk Factors Associated with Abdominal Obesity." *Medical Hypotheses* 44 (1995): 278–286.

McCarty, M. F., and M. Majeed. "The Pharmacology of Citrin." In *Citrin: A Revolutionary, Herbal Approach to Weight Management,* edited by M. Majeed and others, pp. 34–51. Burlingame, Calif.: New Editions Publishing, 1994.

Nomura, F., and K. Chinishi. "Liver Function in Moderate Obesity—Study in 534 Moderately Obese Subjects Among 4,613 Male Company Employees." *International Journal of Obesity* 10 (1986): 349–354.

O'Connor, Deborah L. "Is Optimal Glucose Control Worthwhile?" *Patient Care,* February 15, 1998, pp. 23–24.

Olefsky, J. M. *Current Approaches to the Management of Type-2 Diabetes: A Practical Monograph.* National Diabetes Education Initiative for Health Care Professionals, Professional Graduate Services, 1997.

———. "Pathophysiology of Type-2 Diabetes." *Current Approaches to the Management of Type-2 Diabetes: A Practical Monograph.* National Diabetes Education Initiative for Health Care Professionals, Professional Graduate Services, 1997, pp. 7–14.

Panksepp, J., A. Pollack, R. Meeker, and A. C. Sullivan. "(-)-Hydroxycitrate and Conditioned Aversions." *Pharmacology Biochemistry and Behavior* 6 (1977): 683–687.

Perry, L. M., and J. Metzger. *Medicinal Plants of East and Southeast Asia.* Cambridge, Mass.: MIT Press, 1980, pp. 174–176.

Pullinger, C. R., and G. F. Gibbons. "The Role of Substrate Supply in the Regulation of Cholesterol Biosynthesis in Rat Hepatocytes." *Biochemistry Journal* 210 (1983): 625–632.

Rao, R. Nageswara, and K. K. Sakariah. "Lipid-Lowering and Antiobesity Effect of (-)Hydroxycitric Acid." *Pergamon Journals,* Let., 1988. Abstract.

Rath, M. *Eradicating Heart Disease.* San Francisco: Health Now, 1993.

Schardt, D., and S. Schmidt. "Supplement Watch: Chromium." *Nutrition Action Healthletter,* May 1996, pp. 10–11.

Scoville, B. A. "Review of Amphetamine-like Drugs by the Food and Drug Administration: Clinical Data and Value Judgments." In *Obesity in Perspective: Proceedings of the Fogarty Conference,* pp. 441–443. Washington, D.C.: U.S. Government Printing Office, 1973.

Sener, A., and W. J. Malaisse. "Hexose Metabolism in Pancreatic Islets. Effect of (-)-Hydroxycitrate upon Fatty Acid Synthesis and Insulin Release in Glucose-Stimulated Islets." *Biochimie* 73 (1991): 1287–1290.

Sergio, W. "A Natural Food, the Malabar Tamarind, May Be Effective in the Treatment of Obesity." *Medical Hypotheses* 27 (1988): 39–40.

Silverstone, T. "Drugs, Appetite and Obesity: A Personal Odyssey." *International Journal of Obesity* 16, supplement 2 (1992): S49–S52.

Stock, M. J. "Thermogenesis and Energy Balance." *International Journal of Obesity* 16, supplement 2 (1993): S13–S16.

Sullivan, A. C. "The Influence of (-)-Hydroxycitrate on in Vivo Rates of Hepatic Glycogenesis, Lipogenesis and Cholesterogenesis." *Federation Proceedings* 33 (1974): 656.

———. "Metabolic Inhibitors of Lipid Biosynthesis as Anti-obesity Agents." In *Biochemical Pharmacology of Obesity,* edited by P. B. Curtis-Prior, pp. 311–325. Amsterdam: Elsevier Science Publishers, 1983.

———. "Reactivity and Inhibitor Potential of Hydroxycitrate Isomers with Citrate Synthase, Citrate Lyase and ATP Citrate Lyase." *Tile Journal of Biological Chemistry* 252, no. 21 (1977): 7583–7590.

Sullivan, A. C., and K. Comai. "Pharmacological Treatment of Obesity." *International Journal of Obesity* 2 (1978): 167–189.

Sullivan, A. C., and R. K. Gruen. "Mechanisms of Appetite Modulation by Drugs." *Federation Proceedings*, Part I (1985): 139–144.

Sullivan, A. C., J. G. Hamilton, O. N. Miller, and V. R. Wheatley. "Inhibition of Lipogenesis in Rat Liver by (-)-Hydroxycitrate." *Archives of Biochemistry and Biophysics* 150 (1972): 183–190. Abstract.

Sullivan, A. C., and J. Triscari. "Metabolic Regulation as a Control for Lipid Disorders. I. Influence of (-)-Hydroxycitrate on Experimentally Induced Obesity in Rodent." *American Journal of Clinical Nutrition* 30 (1977): 767–776. Abstract.

———. "Possible Interrelationship Between Metabolic Flux and Appetite." In *Hunger: Basic Mechanisms and Clinical Implications*, edited by D. Novin, W. Wyriwicka, and G. Bray, pp. 115–125. New York: Raven Press, 1976.

Sullivan, A. C., J. Triscari, and L. Cheng. "Appetite Regulation by Drugs and Endogenous Substances." In *Nutrition and Drugs— Current Concepts in Nutrition*, vol. 12, edited by M. Winick, pp. 139–167. New York: John Wiley and Sons, 1983.

Sullivan, A. C., J. Triscari, and K. Comai. "Pharmacological Modulation of Lipid Metabolism for the Treatment of Obesity." *International Journal of Obesity* 8, supplement 1 (1984): 241–248.

Sullivan, A. C., J. Triscari, and J. G. Hamilton. "Hypolipidemic Activity of (-)-Hydroxycitrate." *Lipids* 12, no. 1 (1977): 1–9.

Sullivan, A. C., J. Triscari, J. G. Hamilton, and O. N. Miller. "Effect of (-)-Hydroxycitrate upon the Accumulation of Lipid in the Rat: II. Appetite," *Lipids* 9 (1974): 129–134.

Sullivan, A. C., J. Triscari, J. G. Hamilton, O. N. Miller, and V. R. Wheatley. "Effect of (-)-Hydroxycitrate upon the Accumulation of Lipid in the Rat: I. Lipogenesis." *Lipids* 9 (1974): 121–128.

Sullivan, A. C., J. Triscari, and H. E. Spiegel. "Metabolic Regulation as a Control for Lipid Disorders. II. Influence of (-)-Hydroxycitrate upon Genetically and Experimentally Induced Hypertriglyceridemia in the Rat." *American Journal of Clinical Nutrition* 30 (1977): 777–784. Abstract.

Thom, E. "Hydroxycitrate (HCA) in the Treatment of Obesity." *International Journal of Obesity* 20, supplement 4 (1996): 75. Abstract.

Triscari, J., and A. C. Sullivan. "Comparative Effects of (-)-Hydroxycitrate and (+)-allo-Hydroxycitrate on Acetyl CoA Carboxylase and Fatty Acid and Cholesterol Synthesis in Vivo." *Lipids* 12, no. 4 (April 1977): 357–363.

Voet, D., and J. C. Voet. *Biochemistry*. New York: John Wiley and Sons, 1990.

Wadden, T. A., and A. J. Stunkard. "Psychosocial Consequences of Obesity and Dieting." In *Obesity: Theory and Therapy*, 2d ed. New York: Raven Press, 1993).

Walsh D'epiro, Nancy. "Alarming Diabetes Numbers from the CDC." *Patient Care*, February 15, 1998, p. 18.

———. "Bloodless Monitoring: Coming Soon?" *Patient Care*, February 15, 1998, p. 20.

———. "Of Lost Limbs." *Patient Care*, February 15, 1998, p. 19.

Watson, J. A., M. Fang, and J. M. Lowenstein. "Tricarballylate and Hydroxycitrate: Substrate and Inhibitors of ATP: Citrate Oxaloacetate Lyase." *Archives of Biochemistry and Biophysics* 135 (1969): 209–217.

The Wealth of India (Raw Materials), vol. 4. New Delhi: Council Sci. Ind. Res., 1956, p. 99

Wheeler, Thomas J. "Hydroxycitrate as a Weight Loss Ingredient." Department of Biochemistry, University of Louisville School of Medicine, 1996. Abstract, via Internet.

Zinman, B. "Guidelines for the Management of Type 2 Diabetes." *Current Approaches to the Management of Type-2 Diabetes: A Practical Monograph*. National Diabetes Education Initiative for Health Care Professionals, Professional Graduate Services, 1997, pp. 19–22.

Recommended Reading

Alterman, Seymour L. *How to Control Diabetes*. New York: Ballantine Books, 1996.

American Heart Association. *Your Heart: American Heart Association's Complete Guide to Heart Health*. New York: Simon and Schuster, 1995.

Balch, James F. *Prescription for Nutritional Healing*, 2nd ed. New York: Avery Publishing Group, 1997.

Barnard, Neal. *Eat Right, Live Longer*. New York: Crown, 1995.

Braley, James. *Dr. Braley's Food Allergy and Nutrition Revolution*. New York: Keats Publishing, 1992.

Carlson, Richard. *Don't Sweat the Small Stuff . . . and It's All Small Stuff*. New York: Hyperion, 1997.

Chopra, Deepak. *Ageless Body, Timeless Mind*. New York: Harmony Books, 1993.

Covey, Stephen R. *First Things First*. New York: Simon and Schuster, 1994.

————. *The Seven Habits of Highly Effective People*. New York: Simon and Schuster, 1989.

Diamond, Harvey, and Marilyn Diamond. *Fit for Life*. New York: Warner Books, 1985.

————. *Fit for Life II: Living Health*. New York: Warner Books, 1987.

Greene, Bob, and Oprah Winfrey. *Make the Connection*. New York: New Sage Press, 1997.

Kamen, Betty. *The Chromium Connection: A Lesson in Nutrition*. Novato, CA: Nutrition Encounter, 1996.

Katahn, Martin. *The T-Factor Diet*. New York: W. W. Norton, 1993.

Kelley, David B. *American Diabetes Association Complete Guide to Diabetes*. New York: Bantam Books, 1996.

Klatz, Ronald, and Robert Goldman. *Stopping the Clock: Dramatic Breakthroughs in Anti-Aging and Age Reversal Techniques*. New York: Keats Publishing, 1996.

Larkin, Marilyn. *Redux, the Revolutionary Weight Loss Drug*. New York: Avon Books, 1997.

Lyman, Howard F. *The Mad Cowboy: Plain Truth from the Cattle Rancher Who Won't Eat Meat*. New York: Scribner, 1998.

Marti, James E. *Alternative Health Medicine Encyclopedia: The*

Authoritative Guide to Holistic and Nontraditional Health Practices. Detroit: Visible Ink Press, 1995.

McDougall, John A. *The McDougall Program: Twelve Days to Dynamic Health.* New York: Penguin Group, 1990.

———. *The McDougall Program for Maximum Weight Loss.* New York: Penguin Group, 1994.

Ornish, Dean. *Dr. Dean Ornish's Program for Reversing Heart Disease.* New York: Ballantine Books, 1996.

Ornish, Dean. *Love and Survival: The Scientific Basis for the Healing Power of Intimacy.* New York: HarperCollins, 1997.

Pizzorno, Joseph. *Total Wellness: Improve Your Health By Understanding the Body's Healing Systems.* Rocklin, CA: Prima Publishing, 1996.

Pritikin, Nathan. *The Pritikin Program for Diet and Exercise.* New York: Grosset and Dunlap, 1979.

Pritikin, Robert. *The New Pritikin Program: The Premier Health and Fitness Program for the '90s.* New York: Simon and Schuster, 1990.

Robbins, John. *Diet for a New America.* Walpole, NH: Stillpoint Publishing, 1987.

Ruden, Ronald A. *The Craving Brain.* New York: HarperCollins 1997.

Sauvage, Lester R. *The Open Heart: Stories of Hope, Healing, and Happiness.* Deerfield Beach, FL: Health Communications, 1996.

Slack, Warner V. *Cybermedicine: How Computing Empowers Doctors and Patients for Better Health Care.* San Francisco: Jossey-Bass, 1997.

St. James, Elaine. *Living the Simple Life.* New York: Hyperion, 1996.

———. *Simplify Your Life.* New York: Hyperion, 1994.

Weil, Andrew. *Spontaneous Healing.* New York: Alfred A. Knopf, 1995.

Wurtman, Judith J. *The Serotonin Solution.* New York: Ballantine Books, 1996.

Time Life Books. *Dr. Koop's Self-Care Advisor.* New York: Health Publishing Group, 1996.

———. *The Medical Advisor: The Complete Guide to Alternative and Conventional Treatments.* New York: Time Life Books, 1996.

Vayda, William. *Mood Foods: The Psycho-Nutrition Guide.* Berkeley, CA: Ulysses Press, 1995.

Yanker, Gary, and Kathy Burton. *Walking Medicine.* New York: McGraw-Hill, 1990.

Web Sites

These Web site references are listed in the following format:

- Host—author of site.
- URL address.
- Topic areas.

Alternative Medicine Home Page
http://www.pitt.edu/~cbw/altm.html
Resource for finding information relating to alternative
  medicine.

American Association of Diabetes Educators
http://www.diabetesnet.com/aade.html
Diabetes education and online resources.

American Association of Patients and Providers (AAPP)
http://www.aapp.net
Promotes access to care, affordable care, patient choice and
  medical freedom.

American Diabetes Association (ADA)
http://www.diabetes.org
General diabetes information, state references.

American Family Physician
http://www.aafp.org
General information for diabetes and other health concerns.

American Heart Association
http://www.amhrt.org
Information from the American Heart Association.

American Podiatric Medical Association (APMA)
http://www.apma.org
Podiatry information for healthy foot care.

American Psychological Association (APA)
http://www.apa.com
Information from the APA.

American Society of Bariatric Physicians (ASBP)
http://www.asbp.org
Information and referrals for physicians treating obesity and
    related diseases.

Association of American Physicians and Surgeons (AAPS)
http://www.aapp.net
Promotes freedom in medicine.

BetterHealth USA
http://www.betterhealthusa.com
Information about food allergy blood testing and food sensitivities.

Center for Disease Control and Prevention (CDC)
http://www.cdc.gov/diabetes
Diabetes research information translated for public education.

Children with Diabetes
http://www.childrenwithdiabetes.com
Online service for children and families with type 1 diabetes.

Consumer Information Catalog
http://www.gsa.gov/staff/pa/cic/food.htm
Food and nutrition information from the Consumer
    Information Catalog.

Eli Lilly
http://www.lilly.com/diabetes/
General diabetes information from the Lilly Patient Education
    Program.

Foot and Ankle Web Index
http://www.footandankle.com
General information about healthy feet and resources for foot
  problems.

Health World Online
http://www.healthy.com
General information on health and wellness, nutrition.

HealthComm, Inc.
http://www.healthcomm.com
Information on functional medicine, diabetes, and antiaging
  research.

Health*Max*, Inc.
http://www.healthmax.net
Portal to health and wellness information, programs,
  products, and services.

ImmunoLabs
http://www.immunolabs.com
Information for health care providers about food allergy testing.

Juvenile Diabetes Foundation International (JDF)
http://www.jdfcure.com
Juvenile diabetes educational information.

LifeGuide Monitors—Integ Corporation
http://www.integonline.com
LifeGuide™ bloodless glucose monitoring information.

LXN Corporation
http://www.lxncorp.com
Duet™ fructosamine/glucose monitoring meters.

National Eye Institute
http://www.nei.nih.gov
Information about eyes.

National Institute of Diabetes and Digestive and Kidney Disease (NIDDK)
http://www.niddk.nih.gov
General information on diabetes, digestive, and kidney diseases

National Institutes for Health (NIH)
http://www.nih.gov
Access to the NIH and all the organizations that come under it.

National Network for Health
http://www.nnh.org
Collaborative site for health education.

Online Health Library
http://www.healthfinder.gov
Online health information resources site.

SimpleCare
http://www.simplecare.com
Information on low-cost, cash-based health care resources.

U.S. National Library of Medicine
http://www.nlm.nih.gov
The NIH source for detailed medical information.

Vegsource
http://www.vegsource.org/lyman
A source for vegetarian and vegan information.

World Health Organization
http://www.who.ch
Information on a variety of health topics and statistics.

Worldguide Health and Fitness Forum
http://www.worldguide.com/Fitness/hf.html (be sure to cap the F in Fitness)
Information on anatomy, exercise, and strength training.

Phone Numbers

American Association of Diabetes Educators   800-832-6874
References for people with experience in diabetes education.

American Diabetes Association   800-342-2383
References for diabetes education programs in your area.

Bayer Customer Service   800-348-8100
Information about glucometers and Bayer diabetes products.

Consumer Nutrition Hotline   800-366-1655
Reference for registered dietitians in your area.

Health*Max*, Inc.   206-362-1111
Medical wellness information, programs, products and services.

Index

INDEX